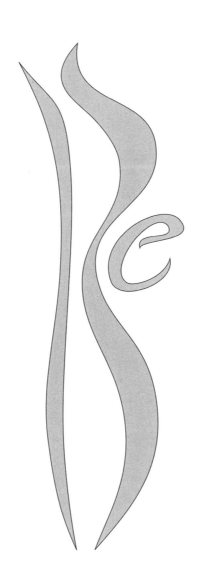

BODY ESTEEM

Weight Loss Through Self-Discovery

Body Esteem ®, Weight Loss Through Self-Discovery
Copyright © 2007 by Sherri Dawson

Published by Luma Publications

To learn more, visit the Body Esteem web site at **www.bodyesteem.com**

The recommendations provided herein are not to be considered medical or psychological advice for the prevention, treatment, or cure of any medical or psychological condition you may currently have or may develop in the future. As with any change in diet and/or exercise, it is important to seek the advice of a medical professional. The intent of the author is only to offer information to help you in your quest for physical fitness and good health.

Printed in the United States of America

ISBN 978-0-9793509-0-0

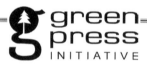
green press
INITIATIVE

Luma Publications is committed to preserving ancient forests and natural resources. We elected to print *Body Esteem, Weight Loss Through Self-Discovery* on 30% post consumer recycled paper, processed chlorine free. As a result, for this printing, we have saved:

11 Trees (40' tall and 6-8" diameter)
4,659 Gallons of Wastewater
1,874 Kilowatt Hours of Electricity
514 Pounds of Solid Waste
1009 Pounds of Greenhouse Gases

Luma Publications made this paper choice because our printer, Thomson-Shore, Inc., is a member of Green Press Initiative, a nonprofit program dedicated to supporting authors, publishers, and suppliers in their efforts to reduce their use of fiber obtained from endangered forests.

For more information, visit www.greenpressinitiative.org

Contents

Foreword

I believe this program is coming at the right moment in history. If you are reading this then it is also the right moment for you.

Eating is a natural function through which you nourish your body and it has a rightful place in your life. You were born knowing when to eat, how much to eat, what to eat and why to eat. Where did you go wrong?

Unfortunately that natural instinct was interfered with from the moment you were born. As a newborn you were probably put on eating schedules that regulated the times you were fed, and what and how much you were supposed to eat.

By the time you were old enough to feed yourself you had already learned that stuffing something into your mouth was a way to handle many of your needs. Then to complicate things more, food began to serve a secondary purpose. It became a replacement for love and affection, and to ease discomfort.

You were given candy as a reward for being good, cookies when you hurt yourself, and an extra portion of dessert if you were "good" and ate everything on your plate.

As you approached adulthood, you were already conditioned to rewarding and comforting yourself with food.

Mass media has also helped create even more misconceptions about the natural place of food in your life.

> "Nothin' says lovin' like something from the oven"
> "Betcha can't eat just one"
> "Bake someone happy"

The TV is constantly telling you to stuff something into your mouth and all will be well.

Through no fault of your own you have been taught to reach for food to satisfy a number of needs that go far beyond your physical need for nutrition.

Overweight, of course is caused by overeating – but more than that – it is a signal from your body telling you that you need to change something in your life.

Body Esteem addresses the real reasons behind your eating patterns. Utilizing the techniques of self-awareness, relaxation, affirmations, and creative visualization, this program takes you on a journey of self-discovery, helping you re-connect with someone you may have lost touch with . . . the inner you. . . that part of you that knows how to listen to what your body wants and nutritionally needs at the time. You will finally be able to open the door and step through into a new body and healthy future.

This program is truly a labor of love. The foundation for Body Esteem began over 20 years ago and has evolved into a comprehensive program after innumerable hours of studying and perfecting the tools that we will share with you.

I formed the ideas behind "Body Esteem" while working with my clients during therapy sessions. Working as a clinical hypnotherapist, I developed techniques that produced dramatic and lasting results for my clients. I found by helping them discover areas of repressed or hidden motivations, they were able to transform their belief system, self-image, and behavior. They were finally able to live a life where they were in control of their responses. As an added bonus, they discovered a new sense of pride in themselves. This program was born out of compassion and the desire to see women truly succeed in their quest for health and self-esteem.

I want to thank Tracie Hinds for her thoughtful contributions to the "Eating for Life" section and Tom Meredith for his expertise in the sound studio. I also want to thank my daughter-in-law Allyne who has provided her insight as a behavioral psychologist and for her support and encouragement to both me and Michael as we worked through the seemingly endless process of getting this book published.

And last, but not least, I want to thank my son and business partner, Michael, for seeing my vision and for pushing me to make it happen. Without his support, encouragement, and artistic contributions to this program, you would not be reading this.

We hope you enjoy and benefit from your journey of self-discovery.

Do it for yourself, you deserve it!

Sherri Dawson

Introduction

Welcome To Body Esteem

If this is your first attempt at losing weight, you're lucky, because you get to do it right the first time. But chances are, you're an "experienced" dieter and have already tried several diets and weight loss methods that produced only marginal or short-term results. Even though you may have resolved to stick to a diet, over and over again, all of your good intentions fell by the wayside long before you reached your goal. You may have lost a few pounds in the process, but you eventually gained them all back, plus a few pounds more.

Have you ever wondered why other people are successful in reaching their goals and maintaining a healthy weight and you are not? If it's any consolation, you are not alone. Overwhelming statistics show that the majority of dieters end up disillusioned and discouraged, short of their goal, weighing more than when they started.

If you were able to lose weight on a diet in the past, obviously the problem was not the diet. What and how much you eat is important, but there's another factor that's more important. In the pages of this workbook you'll discover why your previous attempts were unsuccessful and why this program produces the lasting results you have been seeking.

Your weight is much more than a reflection of the foods you've been eating, it's also a representation of how you feel about yourself and your inner motivations, which are hidden from your conscious mind. In the next few weeks you will uncover and resolve these important and overlooked hidden motivations – an approach, until recently, that has been absent from weight loss programs.

The key to your weight loss is not only WHAT you are eating, but WHY you are eating

The information, written exercises, and recorded programs are designed to help you gain access to your hidden motivations and come to the understanding of how they have been causing you to sabotage your weight loss efforts. You will also learn how to utilize the power of your mind to reinforce your desire and determination to achieving and maintaining your weight goal. Some of the concepts, ideas, and techniques may be new to you, but as you become familiar with them you will see they are the keys to removing the barriers that have prevented your success.

Remember, there are no quick fixes or easy solutions; however, the audio recordings included in this program will make releasing your excess weight easier than it ever has been in the past. As you listen to the recorded programs on a daily basis, you will find your **uncontrollable urges** turning into **automatic healthy responses**, without having to play the willpower game. You will also find you are eating healthier and wanting to exercise, without any conscious effort on your part, as your body, mind and spirit come back into alignment.

If you complete each section as outlined, at the end of this program you will have a greater understanding of yourself and your underlying emotional reasons for overeating. You may also discover a new level of personal confidence and more control over yourself in eating situations. You'll be well on your way to achieving your goal!

You can turn your uncontrollable urges into
automatic healthy responses

One to two pounds a week is a reasonable and healthy rate of weight loss to expect. Typically, you may experience a little more in the beginning, and it may slow as you get close to your weight goal – so don't get discouraged when your rate of loss decreases – it's normal.

When you experience a plateau, remind yourself it is only temporary. If your goal is realistic, you are eating healthfully and following the program, the transformation will come. Nothing positive will come from impatience with your progress. Instead, reaffirm your desire to change, strengthen your belief that you can and will reach your goal, realize that no one else can do it for you, that you alone must do it, and commit to sticking with the program until you reach your goal.

We cannot guarantee you will use this program consistently, or that you will even complete it. We wish we could make that commitment for you – unfortunately we can't. Your success in achieving your weight goal is totally up to you. The best we can do is provide the tools, techniques, and encouragement to make your weight loss efforts successful and permanent.

If you complete this workbook and listen to the recordings as recommended, you will be rewarded with greater self-understanding, confidence, vitality, energy and health. The key is working with the program on a daily basis and taking one step at a time. Your success will be in direct proportion to your degree of commitment. If you make the ultimate commitment, you will be rewarded with a slim and healthy future.

Thank you for honoring yourself by taking the Body Esteem journey.

About the Recorded Programs

This program includes seven carefully designed recorded programs. These recordings are an integral part of the process and are valuable keys to your success. Place them at the top of your daily priority list.

They are designed to clarify, enhance and reinforce the written exercises in the workbook. They utilize positive suggestions, affirmations and creative visualization to help you reach and sustain your weight goal.

As you listen to each recording, you will be guided into a state of peaceful relaxation, after which you will be guided on a journey toward greater self-understanding and health. You will be asked to imagine or visualize yourself in certain situations. These images help reinforce the verbal suggestions and will help you reach your goal more quickly.

Note: Some people are able to mentally create and visualize vivid images in their mind's eye, others only get a sense or feeling of what is being described, while others may only hear what is going on in the environment or situation that is being described. As a test, close your eyes and begin to recall, in your mind's eye, the details in your kitchen – where is your sink, your refrigerator, your range and oven? What colors are your walls, cabinets and counter tops? What do you feel about this room? If there is a window in your kitchen what do you see when you look out from your kitchen? Imagine there are several people in your kitchen having a conversation. What are they talking about? This test will give you an idea of how you will experience the CD's.

In order to receive maximum benefit from these recordings, choose a time and location that will allow you to remain undisturbed for about twenty to twenty-five minutes. Loosen any restrictive clothing. Remove heavy or uncomfortable jewelry, your glasses, and shoes. Find a comfortable position, either sitting or lying down, with your legs and arms uncrossed, your hands resting comfortably in your lap or at your sides. Turn on your player and simply follow the instructions. Using headphones will help your concentration by masking outside sounds and distractions.

As a general rule, listen to the recordings when you are mentally alert and not apt to drift off to sleep; however, several of the recordings are specifically designed so you can listen to them as you go to sleep at night, if you so choose. They allow you to make the choice as to whether you want to awaken at the end of the recording or continue to drift to deeper levels of relaxation leading to your normal, natural, restful state of sleep. It's OK for you to use them at night if you have already listened to them during the day as outlined in the Introduction to each Section. Your mind will hear and reinforce the verbal suggestions while you sleep. This applies to all of the programs except the "Mental Exercises" program. This program is to be used with specific workbook exercises and

CD Recording Titles

CD #1

1. Let's Make An Agreement

2. Imaging Positive Results

3. Set Yourself Free

4. Adventure In Self-Love

CD #2

1. The New You

2. Eliminating Stress

3. Mental Exercises

requires your participation at a more conscious level of awareness.

All of the recordings were designed to be listened to over and over again. They will be as effective a year from now as they are today. You will find them peaceful, calming, repetitive and perhaps somewhat monotonous. Each time you hear the suggestions they become more powerful and eventually will be acted upon automatically without any conscious effort on your part.

When you complete the program, continue to listen to the recorded programs, rotating them as you desire.

If an emergency situation were to arise while you are listening to any of the recordings, you can immediately bring yourself to full alertness in the same way you would if you were engrossed in a daydream.

Whenever you are feeling stressed or overwhelmed, listen to the "Stress Alleviation" program. When your body is in a state of tension, the natural processes of your body are inhibited, and your weight loss will slow or you may even gain weight. Listening to this program will help you deal with your daily stresses in a more positive way.

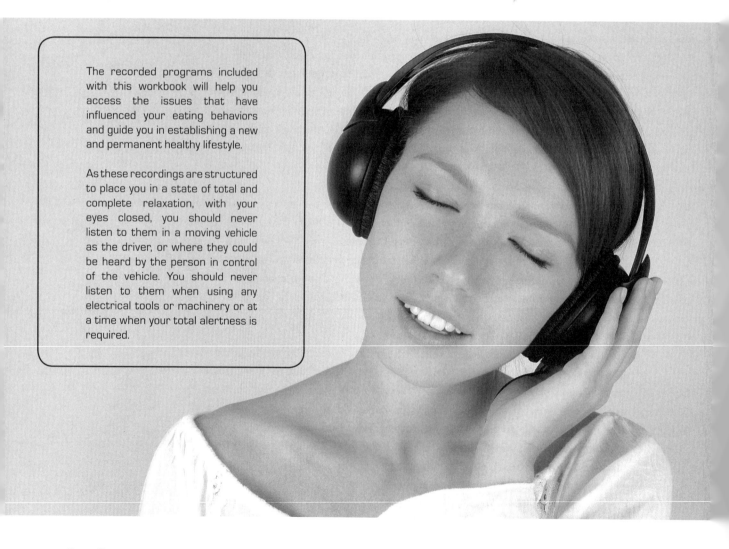

The recorded programs included with this workbook will help you access the issues that have influenced your eating behaviors and guide you in establishing a new and permanent healthy lifestyle.

As these recordings are structured to place you in a state of total and complete relaxation, with your eyes closed, you should never listen to them in a moving vehicle as the driver, or where they could be heard by the person in control of the vehicle. You should never listen to them when using any electrical tools or machinery or at a time when your total alertness is required.

When Should You Start This Program

Choosing the right time to start this program can be almost as important as the program itself. Most of us delay or avoid taking action until we have a good enough reason or we are forced into making a change that we can no longer avoid. Give yourself every advantage by starting with the right mental attitude and sufficient motivation to carry you through to your desired goal.

To help you determine if you are ready to lose weight, evaluate the following statements in relationship to your readiness to starting and following through with this program.

- **I am thinking of losing weight now because someone else wants me to.**

   If your family or friends are putting pressure on you to shed those extra pounds you will probably not have the motivation you need to follow through. Wait until you really want to do it for yourself.

- **I want to lose weight now, even though I have a lot of stress in my life.**

   Postpone starting this program if you have just moved, changed jobs, made some major changes in your life, or there is a crisis in your home. Listen to CD II – Track 3 "***Eliminating Stress***" until you feel your situation has stabilized and you have things under control.

- **I have a special occasion coming up and I need to lose weight fast.**

   This can be a good incentive for getting started . . . however, if you go on a starvation or crash diet to lose your weight too quickly, your body goes into "starvation mode" and lowers your metabolism in an effort to conserve calories, which in turn will stop your weight loss. In addition, when you lose weight too rapidly, your body will use muscle as the primary source of energy. Muscle loss causes a direct decrease in your metabolism and you will find that you will gain weight on fewer calories than before your ill-advised attempt. Try to plan far enough ahead so that you have plenty of time to lose the weight without damaging your body or compromising your health.

- **I am ready to change my health and my appearance, but I'm not sure I have time.**

   We all have busy schedules and it's natural and human to wish to attain your objectives without adding another commitment to your daily routine. If you lived in a perfect world you would have the time you need to do everything you need to do each day. Unfortunately you do not live in a perfect world and you have to make choices. If your health and your appearance is important to you, (and we're assuming it is or you wouldn't be reading this) one of your choices will be to include some time for yourself each day for self-improvement.

Each page of this workbook contains information that is important to your being successful with this program. Every written exercise will bring you closer to uncovering and resolving the real reasons behind your eating behaviors. I know you will be tempted, but PLEASE DON'T SKIP AROUND. This workbook is designed to progress you forward covering a number of different areas and issues. Your readiness for each new Section is based on the information and exercises in the Section you have just completed. Ideally you will physically exercise, complete one reading topic and listen to the CD for the Section you are working in each day. If you are unable to do all three things each day, your order of priority should be: Exercise, Listen to the CD, then the reading or Written Exercises. It's important for you to make this a priority in your life but not to the detriment of your family and/or work commitments. Just make sure you devote some time each day to doing something from this program and you will improve all areas of your life. Move on to the next Section only after you have completed all of the reading and all of the written exercises in each Section.

- **I have accepted I need to make permanent, changes in my eating habits and physical activities in order to reach my weight goal.**

  Far too often, individuals begin a weight loss program with a burst of energy that quickly fades. The result is initial weight loss followed by re-gain. This "up and down Yo-Yo" dieting leads to self-condemnation and a feeling of failure. Are you committed enough to make a sustained effort over an extended period of time? Remember, this program has some tools that will strengthen your desire and commitment to reaching your goal.

- **I am motivated to lose weight but my family is not supporting me.**

  Support and encouragement is important, but it doesn't necessarily have to be from your family. Is there a friend or co-worker who might be interested in starting the program with you? Develop friendships with people who have like interests and will be excited about your successes. Surround yourself with people who care about you and will encourage you to "hang in there" when you reach a plateau or become discouraged. Spend less time with the people who would try to sabotage your efforts as you make positives changes in your life.

- **I don't like to exercise.**

  Exercise is an important part of any weight loss program. You may not like it, but you need to do it.! Don't think of it as work, think of it as your time to play. Find a buddy to exercise with and go "play" together. You will also be less likely to be a "no show" if your exercise buddy is expecting you. You will soon find that you are looking forward to this part of your day.

List in order of importance your reasons for wanting to lose weight.

1. _____
2. _____
3. _____

Are these reasons sufficient to motivate you to following through until you reach your goal?
YES ___ NO ___

Do you think now is the right time for you?   YES ___ NO ___

If your answer is No, what needs to change in order for you to feel you are fully ready to make the commitment to changing your life in a positive way?

_____

_____

Do you have the control to make the changes that will allow you to move forward?   YES ___ NO ___

If your answer is No, who or what does? _____

Why do you not have control over this part of your life? _____

_____

The Importance of Nutrition

What you eat is reflected in your health and appearance and determines the quality of your existence.

Y ou can't live without food – it's necessary for your survival! We all want the same things from food - we want to enjoy the foods we eat and we want the foods we enjoy to nourish our body. Unfortunately, society in the latter part of the twentieth century adopted an ideology of eating based on an economy of time and money. The result was the manufacture and consumption of highly processed, low cost, quick meals. The focus became less on nourishment and more on enjoyment, loading foods full of toxins in the form of fats, sweeteners and preservatives. As a society we are now seeing the effects of an unhealthy lifestyle- a drastic rise in the average weight of women and a substantial increase in diabetes and heart disease.

Our lifestyle has become hurried and stressed. The little time we have for eating has become an opportunity for temporary escapism and overindulgence, as if we could make up for the innumerable hours lost to stress.

This program is focused on empowering you to make-over your body from the inside out. Body Esteem provides you with the bedrock of self-love and understanding upon which you can build a new healthy lifestyle.

The food you eat nurtures your mind and supports the proper functioning of your organs and your physical appearance. By adopting healthy eating as part of your new lifestyle, you will not only achieve your ideal weight, you will discover a number of additional benefits, including: increased energy levels, firmer radiant skin, and the longevity to enjoy your new life!

Your body is unique and it responds to food in its own unique way. You need to determine what is best for your body based on your goals while following certain healthful guidelines. We have included a valuable reference about healthy eating at the back of this book. While we have included the basic tools to get you started on your new relationship with food, it is only the beginning of a journey into a lifetime of health.

Any healthy eating program includes:

True Weight Control Is Not a Diet – It's a Healthier Way of Living

- A balanced diet with a variety of whole foods, that can be purchased at your local supermarket and/or a Farmer's Market

- An intake of food that is adequate in vitamins, minerals and antioxidants

- Drinking 64 oz. of water a day

Any responsible healthy eating plan should be easy to follow, nutritionally sound, and one which allows you a variety of options to satisfy your own food preferences. Following such a plan will create changes in your eating patterns you will want to live with for the rest of your life.

Knowledge is Power

It will be to your benefit to become a student of your body and aware of its nutritional needs and how it responds to the different foods you eat. One of the things most people resist is being told, "You should eat this because it's good for you." But when it's a discovery you make on the path to health, it somehow feels different. By doing a little research of your own, you'll acquire first hand knowledge and feel a real sense of empowerment. An exploration into the world of nutrition can be a wonderful experience that will open you up to the importance of the quality of food that sustains your body. Sources for learning more about nutrition include a qualified dietician, books, your local health food store, and the internet.

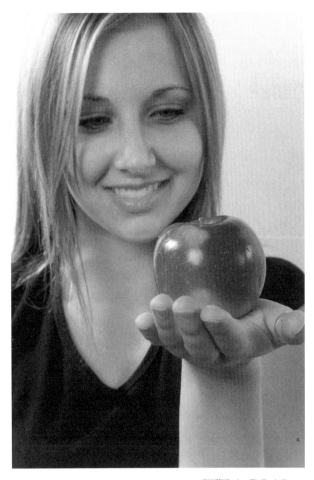

SET A GOAL to eat three balanced meals a day.

One Step At A Time

The process of changing to a healthy lifestyle can be overwhelming, especially if you have been eating foods that are highly processed or refined and are high in saturated fat. Your taste receptors are accustomed, even addicted, to the flavor and taste of fatty and processed foods. You need to retrain your body to appreciate the flavor and texture of whole foods. As you begin to replace the foods you have been eating with the more nutritious natural foods, you will find you are enjoying the new tastes and textures just as much as you enjoyed the foods you were eating before. *The added bonus will be in how much better you look and feel.*

Start With Reading Labels

Read the labels on everything you put in your body, even ones you are accustomed to eating or are your favorites. Look at **all** of the ingredients. How many additional things (artificial color, flavors, sugar or artificial sweeteners, preservatives, fillers) are added to the product that you will now be adding to your body? If you don't know what one of those strange scientific ingredients is, look it up on-line. The internet offers a wealth of information about food and the harmful side effects of many unnatural food additives. You'll be absolutely surprised at the foods the FDA and USDA have approved that pollute your body. You might find yourself wondering just whose interest these government agencies really have in mind . . . is it your health or healthy profits for big business?

When you are comfortable reading labels, begin replacing processed and refined foods with whole foods. **Start to incorporate more fresh fruits, vegetables and whole grains into your meals.** As a general rule, the closer to nature the food is, the more nutritious. Other factors to consider are organic vs. non-organic produce and the antioxidant value of the food.

Begin to consider healthier substitutes for foods you know are unhealthy. Do research on the internet, read books about the benefits of healthy eating. Spend time getting to know the knowledgeable staff at your local health food stores. Browse the ailses and experiment with different kinds of foods. All it takes is a little experience and knowledge to get beyond the "health food=boring food" stigma. Make it an adventure . . . there is a whole new world of tastes to experience.

The entire time you are doing this be aware of how you are feeling. Are you feeling cleaner inside? Do you feel lighter? Do you feel more balanced? Decide what works for you and what doesn't. You know your body better than anyone else and you should become an expert on what your body needs.

Tune into your body and choose a combination of foods that provide the amount of protein, fats, carbohydrates, vitamins and minerals that keep your body functioning at its optimum.

Time to Re-Think The "Diet"

You've probably tried quite a few so called "diets" that guaranteed success.

Maybe you thought, "If only I could have stuck to the diet I would have lost the weight, but instead I gave up, it was just too difficult with my lifestyle or too expensive."

Fad diets, that deny you access to the bounty of food directly from mother nature, potentially compromise your health by denying you the basic nutrition your body needs. This makes it all that much more difficult to follow because your body screams out for nutrients and your soul cries out for enjoyment. It's no secret that balanced eating is the key. Any diet that relies on an extreme approach is not only unhealthy, it's almost impossible for even the most committed person.

Re-define your definition of "Diet" and discover a new found freedom!

The word "diet" originates from the Greek word, *diaita*, which literally means, "manner of living." So rather than thinking of following a "diet" of food restriction, consider it a choice you are making to live a *full and healthy life*.

A healthy diet that will assure a lifetime of success is not about restrictions, it's about the freedom to make informed decisions about the food you put into your body!

Learn "Body Wisdom" by Asking Your Body the Right Questions

How do you feel after you have finished a meal? Some question you may want to ask include:

- Do I feel physically full, but not satisfied?
- Do I feel like I have more energy?
- Do I feel guilty?
- Do I feel sluggish or tired?
- Do I feel lighter?

With the proper knowledge, commitment, and body wisdom, your healthy eating lifestyle will go beyond your need to lose weight. It will support and enhance your beauty, energy, and longevity!

Learn More About Nutrition

Refer to the "Eating For Life" section to provide you with the first steps to adopting healthy eating habits.

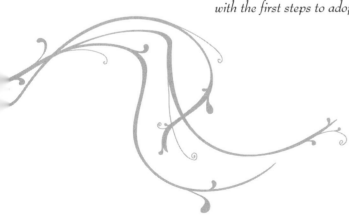

The Value of Exercise

E xercise is an integral part of a healthy lifestyle. It will assist your weight loss efforts by increasing your metabolic rate (how fast you can burn calories), balancing your appetite, and contrary to popular belief, decreasing your needed food intake compared with your former sedentary rate of consumption. Even a moderate amount of exercise will help speed up your ability to burn calories and reduce your craving for food.

A bear, however hard he tries, grows tubby without exercise.

-Winnie the Pooh

As you exercise you are increasing the pumping capacity of your heart, thereby increasing your aerobic (oxygen-using) capacity. The greater your aerobic capacity, the more calories you burn. Any activity that drives your heart rate to about 60-80% of its maximum capacity for any extended length of time, increases your aerobic capacity, thereby increasing your ability to burn calories.

In addition to the metabolic benefits of exercise, your body continues to work for several hours after you have exercised, repairing and regenerating the tissue in the muscles you have used, getting rid of waste products generated by your exercise, and restoring the resting energy supply of glucose and fat in your tissues.

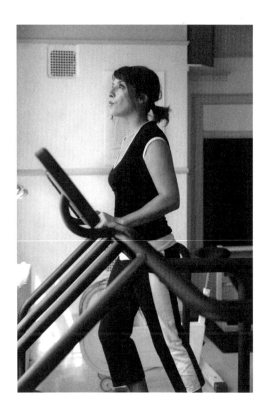

Exercise also provides a healthy release of emotional pressures and tensions, acting as a safety valve, reducing stress and lowering your body's production of cholesterol. As you consistently work with your exercise program you will find you have more energy, greater efficiency, better concentration, less apprehension and better sleep patterns. An added benefit will be a more positive attitude toward life and an increased ability to handle your daily problems more calmly.

Ideally, you want to combine aerobic activity, strength training, and stretching for optimum health. But it's also important to take it one step at a time. Just getting active and finding an activity you enjoy may be an excellent way to begin.

The best type of exercise involves continuous whole-body movement. This type of activity burns the most calories with the least amount of effort. Exercise such as brisk walking, jogging, rebounding, swimming, or biking, that utilize the large muscles in your legs and buttocks to move your body, gives you the biggest payoff for your time and effort.

Walking is possibly the most convenient form of exercise and requires no special equipment, hours, conditions, or previous training. All you really need to invest in is a good pair of supportive shoes and sunblock. It's the best form of exercise to start with because the number of calories you burn is greatest in terms of the effort you expend. If you have not been active recently, it is the safest and quickest way to alter your sluggish metabolism. Walking after eating mobilizes your fat-burning hormones and enzymes and stimulates your muscles to utilize some of the calories you have just consumed.

Smart Steps to Walking

1. *Start slowly and increase your speed* when you feel comfortable at your present pace. Try to walk fast enough to keep your heart rate elevated. You can speed up just by swinging your arms faster, your legs will naturally follow. Caloric expenditure is **62 calories per 100 pounds of body weight per mile traveled** whether you walk, jog or run. For example, if you weigh 150 pounds, you expend 93 calories per mile walked (62 x 1.5). Of course running would burn more calories in the same amount of time because this equation uses distance. The down side of jogging or running can include damage to your joints, a greater chance for muscle injury and may ultimately affect your exercise time because of discomfort you may experience.

2. *Invest in a pedometer and track your steps each day.* The goal is to eventually walk at least 10,000 steps daily. Reaching 10,000 steps can seem intimidating. Think of it as a goal to work toward and in time, you will reach it. The key here is to get out and get moving.

3. *Enjoy your walk.* Notice the trees, fresh air and the abundance of sights and sounds around you. There's a big beautiful world to explore. You can listen to some good tunes or enjoy the company of a friend . . . you can even start an unofficial "girls walking club."

4. *Walk whenever you have a chance.* Intentionally find the furthest distance between two points. Take those extra steps. Park your car at the far end of the parking lot, do as many errands as you can on foot, walk to your neighbor's house rather than calling on the telephone, answer the telephone farthest from where you are, walk into the bank instead of using the drive-in window.

5. *Create goals for yourself.* For example, you could use landmarks . . . "today I will make it to the park." Another kind of goal can be an event to prepare for. **Charity Walks** can be a great goal to work towards. There is nothing quite as rewarding as walking for a cause that is close to your heart. It's a great motivation to get out there everyday and walk a little further, leading up to the day of the charity walk.

Other Forms of Exercise to Explore

Rebounding on a mini-trampoline, ascending a stair climber, or elliptical training on a machine may not be as interesting or enjoyable as a pleasant walk, but it can be done regardless of the weather or time of day. If you find it boring you can watch television or listen to lively music while you are exercising.

Swimming is good exercise because of its lack of stress on your weight-bearing joints. Swimming also can be inconvenient and few people are advanced enough to swim continuously for as long as is necessary to obtain the maximum metabolic benefit. **Aqua Aerobics** is another great way to exercise in the water. The water provides the resistance, yet is much easier on your joints than traditional aerobics.

Bicycling is also inconvenient in most cities and most people do not feel safe riding at speeds that will give the metabolic benefits that are equivalent to walking. Indoor stationary bicycles are an alternative but they can be boring and uncomfortable. *When you feel ready, you can look for a good beginning "spinning" class for a fun, challenging experience on a stationary bike.*

Exercise should never cause you extreme discomfort, especially in your joints. Forget the saying "no pain, no gain". If it hurts, you are exercising incorrectly and should seek the advice of a fitness expert.

Weight training and fitness conditioning are excellent for people who enjoy a challenge. It is a great way to tone, but involves a steeper learning curve and risks injury if unsupervised. It's recommended that you work with a trainer at a gym or with a good video.

There are many **alternative forms of exercise** to choose from including hip-hop dance classes to pilates. Yoga, for example, can offer an amazing connection between the mind and body. Yoga strengthens and lengthens muscles through a series of movements and held "poses." Yoga has increased in recent years in the U.S. and elsewhere because of its ability to center the mind and reduce stress while challenging the body. Breathing is emphasized as a way to calm your mind and increase oxygen intake.

It's important you find an activity you enjoy and can return to consistently.

Explore your local organizations that offer exercise programs. Ask questions about the programs they offer. Exercise experts love to talk about their passion and you may be offered a free class just to see if its the right fit for you.

Videos can be a great way to exercise at home if you are unable to attend classes. Need to hear from an expert, but can't find one near your home, your local library and book stores hold a wealth of information.

Whatever activity you choose - start slowly and go at a comfortable pace. Take the first week to condition yourself and to get over any soreness that might occur before you begin to increase your speed or the duration of activity. Try not to work too hard at first. Going in gung-ho can often result in muscle injuries and can leave you so sore you may not be as motivated the next time you exercise. ***Your breathing should be elevated, but not so hard you are gasping for air.***

Exercise can be fun, relaxing, and an important investment in your health and well-being. Building a better body may start a chain reaction that could improve virtually all areas of your life. There's no better time than now to start a program that can give you a whole new outlook on life.

*Remember to always consult your physician before beginning a new exercise program.

A Few Tips To Get You Started

One of the key elements to achieving your ideal body is to increase your daily activity. Incorporate the following into your daily routine whenever you can.

Enjoyment
Choose a form of exercise you enjoy. Don't think of it as work, think of it as your time to play. Engage in activities that use the large leg muscles such as walking, rebounding or dancing!

Sleepy? Take A Walk
When you feel like napping – TAKE A WALK. If you feel sleepy shortly after a meal, look at what you ate. You may have eaten too much and/or it may have been comprised of too many carbohydrates and sweets and too little protein. If you feel run down at the end of the day, the reason could be psychological rather than physical. After working all day, when the end of the day comes you instinctively relax and let down. This emotional release has a way of translating itself into inactivity. Your real need at this time is for a new surge of activity to revitalize your mental outlook.

Climb Stairs
Whenever you can, climb stairs. Climbing burns twice as many calories as walking on the level. Your body gets a cardiovascular workout after four flights. Climbing two steps at a time burns even more calories. If you live in a two-story house, get into the habit of using the upstairs bathroom.

Weighing In For Results

Your weight will vary from day to day and from morning to evening. Although your scales can serve as a practical gauge of increases and decreases in body weight, they do not change the shape of your body nor are they accurate reflections of your body fat.

The numbers on your scale <u>only</u> indicates total body weight, which includes:
   1) Body fluids
   2) Lean muscle tissue, which weighs more than fat
   3) Body fat stores
   4) Contents of your stomach and intestines

- Weigh yourself on the first morning you begin this program.
- Be consistent. After your first weigh-in, weigh yourself only **ONCE A WEEK** on the **SAME DAY** and preferably at the **SAME TIME** each week.
- Always weigh yourself the first thing in the morning, without clothing, with an empty bladder and before you have eaten.

Normal daily fluctuations in weight and temporary plateaus will discourage you if you weigh too often. Besides, the scale only measures your total body weight, it doesn't tell you about your fat content (unless it is a new one with this feature), muscle content, or metabolism.

If the scales don't show a substantial weight loss, don't get discouraged, you may be losing more inches than fat. You may be building muscle from the exercise you are doing. Remember, muscle weighs more than fat. Rely on your measurements to determine if you are moving toward your goal. **Do the numbers on the scale really matter that much if you look and feel good?**

The following body measurements should be taken with a cloth measuring tape <u>once every two weeks</u>.

- *Chest* - measure around your chest at the nipple line.
- *Waist* - measure around your waist at the level of your belly button.
- *Hips* - measure around your hips 7" below your waistline.
- *Upper thigh* - measure around the uppermost part of your thigh.
- *Mid thigh* - measure around your thigh, halfway between your knee and the uppermost part of your leg.
- *Arm* - measure halfway between your shoulder and elbow, with your arm hanging down naturally.

* Talk to a professional, such as a dietician or a physician, when determining your weight goal, he or she can help you set a goal that is reasonable, healthy and safe.

Weight and Measurement Chart   Date Started   /   /

	Weight	Bust or Chest	Waist	Hips	Right Upper Thigh	Left Upper Thigh	Right Mid Thigh	Left Mid Thigh	Right Arm	Left Arm
Week 1										
Week 2										
Week 3										
Week 4										
Week 5										
Week 6										
Week 7										
Week 8										
Week 9										
Week 10										
Week 11										
Week 12										
Week 13										
Week 14										
Week 15										
Week 16										
Week 17										
Week 18										
Week 19										
Week 20										
Week 21										
Week 22										
Week 23										
Week 24										

Weight and Measurement Chart

You must resist the urge to weigh every day.

My Picture
Before

You may have some resistance to having your picture taken or placing a full body picture of yourself in this space. This "before" picture is important because in a few weeks you will be able to use it as a comparison to readily see how far you have come.

My Picture Tips:

Try to take the pictures with the same camera, same lighting conditions and the same distance away.

Use a 4x6 photo.

Date _____   Weight Today _____   My Weight Goal* _____

My Picture
After

Notice the change that has come in just a few weeks!

Beyond the weight loss, you may also see a change in the expression on your face and an extra twinkle in your eyes. Your skin may appear healthier and your face younger.

If you haven't reached your goal by the end of this program, don't worry, changes take time. Look at the changes that have occurred and allow them to inspire you to continue your healthy lifestyle for the rest of your life!

You have a lifetime of health and happiness to enjoy your new body.

Date _____   Weight Today _____

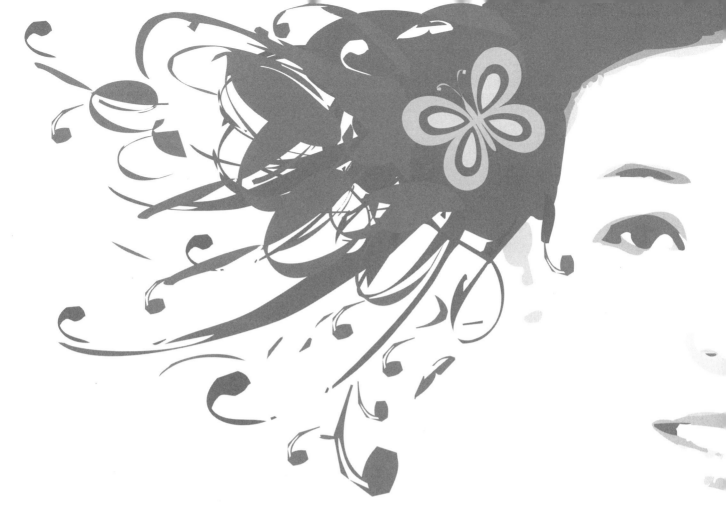

Getting Started

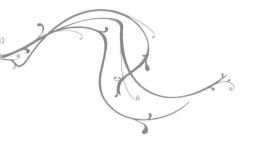

Getting Started

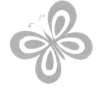

This is where you begin your journey. As with many important journeys, you must commit yourself to the challenge ahead and study how you will succeed.

The first step on your new path is to make the commitment to a healthy lifestyle. The "Weight Loss Agreement" on page 26 is the physical companion to the "*Let's Make an Agreement*" recording. Signing this contract with yourself signifies a deeper commitment to your goal. We ask you to re-read your agreement daily and listen to the "*Let's Make an Agreement*" recording every day while working in this section. You may also listen to this recording when you go to sleep at night. This repetition will strengthen your commitment and help insure your success.

Your next step will be recording your food intake and understanding the role your emotions play in your eating patterns. Learning to distinguish your desire to eat when it is motivated by an emotional need could be the first key to gaining insight into your unhealthy eating behavior.

Food journaling is a proven method that will allow you to look at the amount and quality of the food you are eating.

By understanding your patterns and the areas for improvement, you will be able to better plan your meals.

You will also look at some potential traps you may encounter along the way. Learning to recognize them will help you avoid pitfalls you may have experienced in the past.

The "Mental and Written Exercises" in this workbook are important tools for insight and will greatly aid in your success. Be sure to complete *"Mental Exercise 1."* Doing this will alert you to the obstacles you may have to overcome to reach your goal.

The road to success may not always be easy, but this program will help empower you to find your strength within to achieve your dreams of health and beauty.

Weight Loss Agreement

I acknowledge that I am a unique individual with the power and the ability to create my own destiny.

I acknowledge that I am responsible for gaining the weight and I now accept the responsibility for releasing it.

I am making a fresh, new start. In the near future, I will allow myself to obtain, maintain and sustain my ideal weight. I want this, I know I am capable of achieving it, and I expect to succeed.

It has taken me time to gain the weight and I now realistically set my goals for releasing it. I am committed to reaching the weight goal I have set for myself in a safe and healthy manner. I truly believe I am capable of accomplishing my goal. I have the desire, determination and self-discipline to stick with it until my goal of a healthy, attractive body is my reality.

I now consciously and subconsciously accept my weight goal as one of my most important and desirable goals.

I am persistent, yet gentle with myself as I move toward the achievement of my goal. I am releasing all negative and undesirable attitudes I have about myself, as well as the negative attitudes I have about others. I am committed to following the section plans, knowing as I take action, change takes place.

I am restoring a sense of well being and harmony for myself on the mental, emotional, physical, and spiritual levels, so change can take place, bringing into balance my entire being.

I am creating a positive reality for myself and I am proud of myself. I am doing this for myself because I love myself and I deserve it. I am interested in my future for I am going to spend the rest of my life there.

I enter into this Agreement with myself, for myself,
on this_____day of_____, 200_____.

_____
Signature

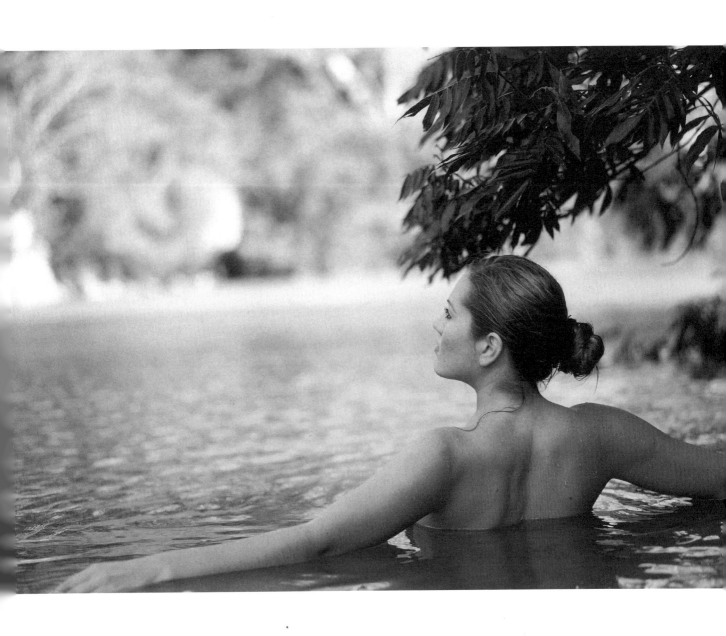

The Importance of Food Journaling

You may already be familiar with food journals or this may be your first experience with one. If you have kept a food journal in the past you already know it can be a tedious exercise, but nothing will make you more aware of unhealthy eating like writing down your every sip, taste and slip-up on a food journal. At the end of the week you will know exactly what and how much you have been eating each day and it will help you realistically look at some things about your eating habits that you may have been ignoring.

And here are some other reasons for you to do a journal:

- Charles Stuart Platkin, founder and director of the Institute for Nutrition and Behavioral Sciences says "keeping a record of everything you eat and the reason you are eating is critical when you are trying to identify your emotional eating behaviors. If you chart what and when you're eating along with how you feel, you should start seeing patterns."

- The National Weight Control Registry - in an ongoing research project that tracks over 3,000 people who have lost an average of 66 pounds and kept if off for over five years - found that keeping a food journal is one of the strategies used by the majority of all highly successful dieters.

- Betty Kovacs, M.S. RD, Nutrition Coordinator of St. Luke's Roosevelt Obesity Research Center in New York City, states "keeping a food record is the one thing I can say has proven to work for every single person."

- A breakthrough study conducted at OSF-St. Francis Medical Center in Illinois found that whenever a celebration week cropped up, non-journal dieters gained five times the weight they'd lost the previous week, while those who did keep diaries actually lost weight! Journaling just five days a week has been proven to *double* weight loss.

For this exercise to be of value, YOU MUST CONTINUE TO EAT AS YOU NORMALLY DO for one more week. You must record EVERYTHING you put into your mouth - including that one bite of ice cream you snitched when you dished it up for your kids. Even that one bite contains calories and provides insight into your eating patterns. For example, look at how fast calories add up when you have the six potato chips, a handful of popcorn, four french fries, one bite of a candy bar, two swallows of cola, and the hard corner of a brownie. You may have added several hundred calories to your daily total with those unhealthy "little" indulgences.

Recording the number of calories for each meal, while helpful, is not required in our exercises. For now, your time will be much better spent on educating yourself about proper nutrition and balanced eating.

Eventually, you may want to incorporate calorie counting into your food journals. To start, you might find it helpful to know just how many calories are in the fast food you are eating. You will probably be shocked, particularly if you have been "having fries with that . . ." After you recover from the shock, you probably will be motivated to cut out a significant number of calories just by making more conscious meal decisions or by preparing your own meals at home.

Since one pound of fat equates to approximately 3,500 calories, to lose one pound a week you need to consume approximately 3,500 fewer calories per week. **You can do this by reducing your daily calorie intake by 500 calories per day.** Remember, one to two pounds a week is a reasonable and healthy goal.

Food journaling is also an excellent tool to help you become aware of the **quality of the food** you are eating. It will help illuminate your unhealthy eating patterns and some of the reasons for these patterns.

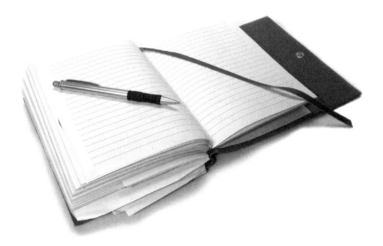

Body Esteem is about self-knowledge and the power to determine the quality of your life. Food journaling is an important tool to have with you on this journey.

Note: You will find 7 days of Food Journal pages in the "Forms" section at the back of this workbook.

Successful Food Journaling Keys

Key #1: Concentrate on Nutrition

Start thinking about the nutritional value of the foods as you record them. Also record approximately how much you ate. Analyze each meal and make notations of what foods you could substitute to support your weight loss and increase you level of health and vitality.

Key #2: Stay Hydrated

Be sure to record everything you drink, including your water intake. All functions within the body require the presence of water. A well hydrated body enables these functions to occur quickly and efficiently. Drinking your recommended daily intake of H2O will also assist you in losing weight, as it stimulates your metabolism to work more efficiently and results in less water retention. Drinking water before, during, and after exercise will keep your energy levels high and help recovery after a workout. Water also releases toxic waste products from your cells, helps joint pain and improves your skin.

Eating fruit high in water content is an excellent way to augment your liquid hydration. Most fruits are low in calories and deliver naturally occurring vitamins and minerals to your body.

Note: If you have kidney problems or other conditions where fluid intake needs to be limited, seek advice from your doctor before changing your water drinking habits.

*Be willing to go through the process
and you will produce the results*

Key #3: Recording Physical Hunger

It will also be helpful for you to rate your **physical** hunger on a scale of 1-10 before each meal.

As you record your food intake in the journal you will become aware of your eating patterns and snacking habits and you will become more aware of how your body responds to the foods you eat.

Benefits of Recording Physical Hunger

- You will discover certain foods may satisfy your taste buds, but leave you feeling hungry before you have finished your meal.

- You will develop an increased awareness of the foods that meet your nutritional requirements, giving you energy to carry out your daily activities and stabilizing your mood throughout the day.

- You will learn to distinguish between the sensations that are prompted by actual physical hunger and those stimulated by an unconscious need.

When you are reaching for a snack, become aware of why you are eating at this particular time.

- Are you mindlessly following commercial programming that has created emotional connections with certain foods?

- Are you really hungry or just craving something salty or sweet?

- Are you eating out of habit such as eating a snack at break time?

- Do you feel like you just need something to chew on?

- Are you just being sociable?

- Are you eating, just because it's there?

Key #4: Record Your Emotions

You should also record your **mood**. Circle whether you were angry, content, depressed, frustrated, happy, sad, stressed, or tired. Because much of your eating may be to satisfy emotional needs, learning to distinguish between the sensations prompted by actual physical hunger and those stimulated by a psychological or emotional need is an important step on your path to taking back the control food has had over you.

Become aware of what you are feeling.

- Are you angry, anxious, lonely, depressed, feeling empty inside, under stress, rewarding yourself, or responding to an outside stimulus such as an ad on TV?

- Did eating make you feel better?

Record these feelings in your journal as well. By the end of the week you will begin to see some patterns developing that will give you some insight into your unconscious motivations.

Key #5: Record Your Eating Patterns Until Healthy Eating Becomes Automatic

It is strongly recommended you continue to record your food intake at least through the end of this program. Hopefully you will find it has been beneficial and you will want to continue until you reach your weight goal. Keeping a food journal until you reach your goal will alert you to changes in your calorie intake so you can make adjustments immediately before they show up as unwanted pounds on your scale.

Just a reminder - **your success will be *in direct proportion to the amount of effort and commitment you put into this program*** - so think about how successful you want to be before you throw your future away.

NOTE: It will be helpful to carry a small journal with you to record your food intake when you are away from home. It's too easy to forget exactly what and how much you ate and drank if you wait till the end of the day to complete your food journal.

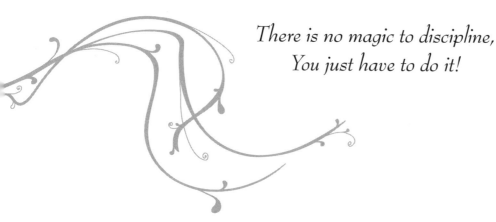

There is no magic to discipline,
You just have to do it!

Emotional Eating

The feelings you perceive as hunger are stimulated not only by a physical need for food but are also activated by the mental, emotional, social and spiritual aspects of your personality as well.

True hunger is motivated by a physical need for food. After you have eaten a meal and satisfied your nutritional requirements you usually will not experience the physical need for food for another four to six hours. A true "physical hunger" feeling lasts only a short time before disappearing and is recognizable by sensations of faintness, loss of concentration and other physical symptoms.

Emotional hunger, on the other hand, appears when your mind reaches out for food. It is stimulated by your thoughts, feelings, proximity to food, habits, and practically anything you have learned to associate with food.

It is important for you to learn to differentiate when your eating is motivated by a physical need for food and when it results from an internally triggered desire to eat as a response to totally external events.

You can train your mind and emotions to work for you, not against you

Keeping an emotional eating diary, in which you record the feelings and emotions surrounding your eating activities, which occur outside of normally scheduled meal times, will bring you face to face with your emotional eating habits. This diary is one of the steps to becoming aware of your feelings about food and the purpose it serves for you.

For this exercise to be effective you need to list **when**, **what** and **why** you ate. Were you angry, frustrated, bored, nervous, upset, lonely, anxious, or sad? Were you celebrating good news, rewarding yourself, relaxing after a hard day, postponing a chore you dislike, watching television or reading a good book?

As you record your emotional eating in the diary you will begin to recognize the unconscious patterns emerging. Once you are aware, you can start to choose alternative activities and change your uncontrollable urges into automatic healthy responses.

Complete **PART I** of the **EMOTIONAL EATING DIARY** when you feel a strong urge to eat and know you are not in physical need of food.

If, after getting in touch with your feelings, you still go ahead and eat, complete **PART II** of the diary when you have finished eating.

NOTE: You will find more "Emotional Eating Diary" forms in the "Forms" section at the back of this workbook.

Emotional Eating Diary

Day of Week _____ Time _____ **Food Wanted** _____

Part 1 - Emotions Before Eating

Is this food really necessary? YES ___ NO ___

How long has it been since you last ate? _____

Why do you want this particular food?
Look ___ Smell ___ Taste ___ Feel ___ Other ___

What emotional need or feeling are you trying to satisfy? _____

What are your thoughts at this time? _____

What triggered this need for food? Could you satisfy your need in another way? YES ___ NO ___
How? _____

Part 2 - Result After Eating

Did you eat to satisfy an emotional rather than a physical need? YES ___ NO ___
If yes, why did you eat? _____

How could you change that response in the future? _____
_____

Did food satisfy your need? YES ___ NO ___
If no, why not? _____

Potential Pitfalls

We are all aware of the usual diet traps: the cookies you bought "for the kids," the tortilla chips at the Mexican restaurant, the birthday party with all of the foods you have been trying to avoid. There are a number of other things that can cause even your best intentions to fall by the wayside. Be sure to avoid the following pitfalls on the way to your goal.

Wanting to Lose Weight too Quickly

We've all been tempted, and perhaps have even given in to the ads:

"Lose Weight Fast"
"I Lost 60 pounds in 45 Days"
"Lose Up to 30 Pounds in 30 Days."

We know you are anxious to get thinner, but please beware of these claims for quick weight loss. If you read the fine print in the ads they usually state "these results are not typical." The government has issued warnings to many companies not to use deceptive advertising, but we continue to see a flood of false claims in magazine ads, television and especially on the internet.

In any case, losing weight too quickly is damaging to your health and usually is not long lasting. Whatever strategy you choose, make sure it's realistic and incorporates a balanced eating plan, exercise and habits you can live with the rest of your life.

Your weight loss may not be consistent from week to week. Even if you have been eating a calorie-managed diet and exercising consistently, sometimes your scale won't reflect your efforts immediately. Be patient during this time and focus on the positives – you're eating better, you're exercising and you're improving your health . . . it will all pay off, just hang in there! If you are consistently following the program there are many changes taking place that haven't manifested yet at the physical level.

The speed of your weight loss will depend on your percentage of body fat, quality of food, number of calories consumed and number of calories burnt daily. One to two pounds a week is a realistic goal for most people, but you should check with a qualified health professional to determine the rate that is best for you.

The Sweet Tooth

We are born liking the sensation of sweetness. Sweetness can be a sensory cue for energy to fuel metabolic needs and physical activity. Foods that are naturally sweet, such as fruit and breast milk, contain important nutrients to support health. Sweetness is universally regarded as a pleasurable experience. It's no wonder that the desire for sweets is a difficult area to modify in a person's behavior.

Skipping sweets when you are trying to lose weight seems to be one of the cardinal rules of dieting. You might feel like you are depriving yourself of a basic simple pleasure, but denying yourself sweets when you're trying to control your weight can backfire, causing you to go on a sweets binge. You do not have to deprive yourself of sweets, you just need to be committed to creative new alternatives to satisfy your craving for sweets. Natural, low glycemic alternatives available at your health food store might be just the solution. These include sweeteners such as Agave Nectar and Stevia. (You can lean more about these wonderful products in the "Eating for Life" section at the back of this book.)

If you do go on a binge, don't beat yourself up over it and don't use it as an excuse to blow the whole program. Just get back on track and don't make it a habit. As you eliminate unhealthy, calorie loaded sweets from your daily eating plans, you will likely find you are craving them less and less.

Snacking

Snacking has long been a no-no for dieters. After all, how can you lose when you're eating all the time? However, planned snacking actually helps manage your appetite. Eating a low calorie, filling and nutritious snack mid morning and late afternoon will insure you won't be ravenous and overeat at meal times. Eating more often also helps you burn more calories and fat by maximizing the time your metabolism works at peak performance. If you are losing slowly or have reached a plateau, try dividing your daily intake into 3 meals and 2 snacks per day.

Making Others Needs More Important Than Your Own

Being selfless could be preventing you from losing weight. If you spend most of your life giving to others and never taking time for yourself you may feel put upon and resentful at some level. Is eating the only nice thing you are doing for yourself? Give yourself permission to do what you need to do for yourself so resentment doesn't get in the way of reaching your weight goal.

Believing the Celebrity That Says It Will Work For You

Just because it worked for someone else, doesn't mean it will work for you. It doesn't matter what beautiful star appears in the ads to inspire you, it's your body and your future. Chances are they had an army of trainers, consultants and chefs, a diet food or exercise product to insure they would be successful. Remember, if they are advertising a product, there's a good chance they are being paid to do it. More likely than not, your team will be your family and friends, some of whom may not support your new healthy lifestyle.

While role models can be a source of inspiration, the true fire that lights your way on this journey must come from within.

Sweating With An Audience

If you are embarrassed to exercise and "glisten" in front of strangers, joining a gym probably is not going to be comfortable for you. You may do better working out to a video at home until you feel ready to join the masses at the gym.

Keep in mind, working out at home requires a lot of self-motivation and determination. Try to create a weekly schedule for yourself that you follow. Mix things up every once in a while by trying new styles and trainers to keep things fresh and interesting.

Skipping Meals

No weight-loss plan ever works unless you take in fewer calories than you burn each day, but slashing calories drastically never works in the long run either. Skipping meals causes your body to gain weight over the long haul – even if you aren't eating more than you'd have eaten if you ate three meals a day. Why? Because, just like when you go on a super-low-calorie diet, you body adapts to being starved by conserving more calories as fat.

Giving Up

Whatever you do, don't give up! The one difference between yo-yo dieters and the people who lose weight and keep it off is . . . successful dieters stick with the program through the good and the bad days. Just stay focused on your goal, no matter what. If you backslide (and we all do), just get back on track and keep going. Be consistent and the results will come!

Understanding Your Metabolism

The word "Metabolism" refers to all of the biochemical processes through which the food you eat is broken down and its nutritional components transformed for use in rebuilding tissue, constructing your various hormones and enzymes, supplying the energy you need to move your body, and maintaining your vital functions. In other words, your metabolism is all the things your body does to change the nutrients in food into the form your body needs to stay alive!

Your "Basal Metabolism Rate" or BMR is the minimum amount of energy required by your body when it is at rest to maintain its essential vital functions. You may have a very efficient metabolism, which means from the moment digestion begins everything is done with as little wasted energy as possible. Your body does its work so efficiently there are many more calories left over to go into your "fat banks" for storage.

You may have been born with an efficient metabolism, but its also possible you have eaten in a way that changed your perfectly normal metabolism into a "thrifty" one. If you have gone on low calorie diets in an attempt to control your weight you may have changed your already frugal metabolism into an even more thrifty one. You actually gave your body practice on how to eat less and weigh more.

Your body kicks into "starvation mode"
and lowers your metabolism every time
you go on a starvation or crash diet

Our primitive ancestors didn't have the mass quantities of food available like we have today. During times of famine and starvation, their bodies became programmed to slow down metabolism and conserve every calorie in order to survive. That programming hasn't changed. When you go on a low calorie diet, your body doesn't understand you wish to look and feel better, it thinks you are about to starve it. It compensates by cutting back on its metabolic needs by as much as 35 to 45%. Having this trait was great when primitive man was faced with an uncertain food supply, but in our society, with its abundance of food, it's unnecessary. We have to learn how to achieve the results we want without threatening our body.

Eliminate the idea that a "Crash Diet" will help you achieve your goal more quickly. It may be tempting and may seem like it's working, but you will only be sabotaging yourself. When you cut calories drastically your metabolic rate slows down and hits bottom in three to seven weeks. At this point there may be little difference between your restricted intake and your lowered metabolic needs. In addition, when you lose weight too rapidly, your body uses muscle tissue as a primary source of energy. Losing muscle causes your metabolism to decrease even more.

If you get discouraged and deviate from your diet or return to your former intake pattern, weight gain will occur with fewer calories than it previously took to maintain your higher weight. Talk about frustration!

Your metabolic rate will turn on again and start to rise as you begin to eat more, but it may not return to near normal until you have regained a good portion of the weight you have lost. If you eat again exactly at your pre-diet level, you will end up gaining several additional pounds.

In order to improve your metabolism it is important to choose a program that is nutritionally balanced, one that destroys fat rather than muscle and includes an exercise plan to stimulate your metabolism. The best way to determine the ideal caloric intake for your particular body is to consult with a qualified health professional.

What you do to your body today determines your quality of life tomorrow

Mental and Written Exercise Instructions

Your weight is much more than a reflection of the foods you have been eating. It also represents how you feel about yourself, your unconscious motivations (childhood and cultural programming) and established eating habits as a result of your lifestyle.

It's possible your weight is the result of one or more experiences you've blocked from your conscious memory. You may have had an experience at a very early age that you are not aware of at your conscious level of awareness. Perhaps it was too physically painful and/or emotionally traumatic, and you supressed it. These suppressed memories can control the way your mind and your body respond to food.

Undoubtedly you will find some of the exercises in this workbook difficult. It's important to your future success that you push yourself beyond your comfort zone and do your best to complete each exercise. They are designed to help you gain insight and understanding into your motivations and eating patterns.

There are no right or wrong answers to the questions in the mental and written exercises in this workbook. In order for them to be of value, you must answer them as honestly and completely as you possibly can. Become aware of any feelings of nervousness in relationship to particular questions. A certain amount of apprehension is normal when you are confronting the new and unknown. If you experience more than a normal amount of anxiety, this could mean you have suppressed an unpleasant experience or emotion connected to the question. Be aware of the times when you want to answer one way . . . but a nagging little voice inside of you is saying something else. Trust your inner voice, for that is where your true awareness will come from. Many times it will be giving you insight into areas of your past you may have forgotten or haven't wanted to confront.

What will happen as you start to uncover and acknowledge these experiences, feelings, and emotions? You will begin to feel stronger and less like a victim. You will feel more positive about your life and you will find your relationship with food changing in a more healthy direction. These changes may come quickly or they may come slowly over a period of time. With patience, courage and dedication, you will be amazed at the powerful insights that will surface.

As you begin to use food for nourishment rather than to meet emotional or unconscious needs your body will begin to reshape itself without conscious effort on your part.

NOTE: While using the **"Mental Exercises"** recordings in this program you may encounter blocked or forgotten experiences that are upsetting, uncomfortable, or cause you to become very emotional. If this happens it is a good thing because it means you may have gotten in touch with the root cause of your weight problem.

IMPORTANT . . . PLEASE NOTE

If you are having trouble processing the information and your emotional stability is being affected you should discontinue using the "Mental Exercises" recordings immediately and consult a professional counselor who can help you uncover and resolve the experiences you encountered. Discuss this program with your counselor and if they have no objections, continue with the daily reading and the other recorded programs. They will work as a valuable supplement to your counseling sessions.

MENTAL EXERCISES RECORDING

This recorded program is designed to help you gain access to the information stored in your subconscious mind. This information is important because it will help you understand the real reasons you are unable to attain and maintain your ideal weight. Be aware that sometimes the answers you receive may not be what you expect, or even want to acknowledge. Be as open as you can to this new information. Only by uncovering the true reasons behind your overweight will you be free to become the slim, healthy, beautiful person you desire to be.

Choose a time and location where you can be undisturbed for at least 20 minutes. If possible have your CD player within easy reach so you can pause it when instructed to do so during the exercise.

Listen to CD II – Track 3 and mentally ask yourself the following questions when instructed to do so. **Trust the first answer that comes into your mind** and write it in the space provided.

Mental Exercise 1

These questions and statements will alert you to the adjustments you will need to make and the obstacles you will have to overcome to reach your weight goal. Knowing these ahead of time will help you plan for dealing with them as you encounter them.

What made me decide at this time to change my appearance and my life? _____

_____

Looking ahead to the next few weeks and months, is it going to be difficult for me to achieve my goal? YES ___ NO ___

What adjustments am I going to have to make in order to reach my goal? _____

_____

Are the results going to be worth the adjustments I will have to make? YES ___ NO ___

What is the biggest obstacle I will have to overcome? _____

How will I conquer it? _____

_____

Who will support me the most when I feel discouraged? _____

What will other people do to try and sabotage my efforts? _____

_____

How will I handle them? _____

What will I do in an attempt to sabotage myself? _____

How will my life change as I move toward my goal? _____

_____

How will my life change after I have reached my goal? _____

_____

Can I live with the changes? YES ___ NO ___

Will anyone be hurt by my being slim? YES ___ NO ___

If yes, who and how?_____

_____

How will I handle their feelings? _____

What advice would be helpful to me now that I have made the commitment to becoming slim?

_____

_____

 Turn your CD player back on and relax as you listen to the suggestions that will assist you in reaching your weight goal.

Read over the questions and your answers in "Mental Exercise 1" and answer the following questions.

Before doing this exercise had you given any thought to the adjustments you will have to make to achieve your goal?   YES ___   NO ___

Will this awareness help you when you have to make adjustments in order to insure that you do achieve your goal?   YES ___   NO ___

Did the questions allow you to look at your commitment to releasing your excess weight from a different perspective?   YES ___   NO ___

Are you more aware now of the obstacles you may face in achieving your goals?   YES ___   NO ___

Will you be able to overcome the obstacles you encounter?   YES ___   NO ___
If NO, why not?   _____

How can you use the knowledge you gained from your answers to help you overcome the opposition you may face from people who would rather not see you reach your goal?

_____

_____

_____

Wrap-Up

CONGRATULATIONS – YOU HAVE COMPLETED "GETTING STARTED."

Every journey begins with the first step. Your first step was when you decided to purchase this book. At that point you made a commitment to changing your life. That initial commitment helped you continue through the Introduction and completion of this section. In the process you may have encountered new information and new concepts that will support you as you continue your journey to your goal, as well as reinforcing activities and behaviors that are already positive influences in your life.

If you haven't lost any weight, don't get discouraged, you are just getting started. It takes time for your mind and body to realize that you are making some changes in your life. They'll catch up shortly.

Food Journals – a pesky exercise that can also be an eye-opening experience. If you completed the food journals and recorded everything you ate, you are becoming more aware of your food choices. That awareness is one of the first steps to changing the role that food plays in your life.

As you continue on your journey, become aware of times when you are sabotaging yourself, and ask yourself, "why am I doing this to myself?" Don't be afraid to search for the real reasons behind your behavior. Remember "knowledge is power!" and it will help you gain back control over your life.

Every positive thought or action you experience is a plus and indicates you are beginning to make your health and your appearance a priority. If you haven't already done so, reinforce your desire, determination and commitment to achieving your weight goal and to continuing on your journey to becoming the woman you have always wanted to be.

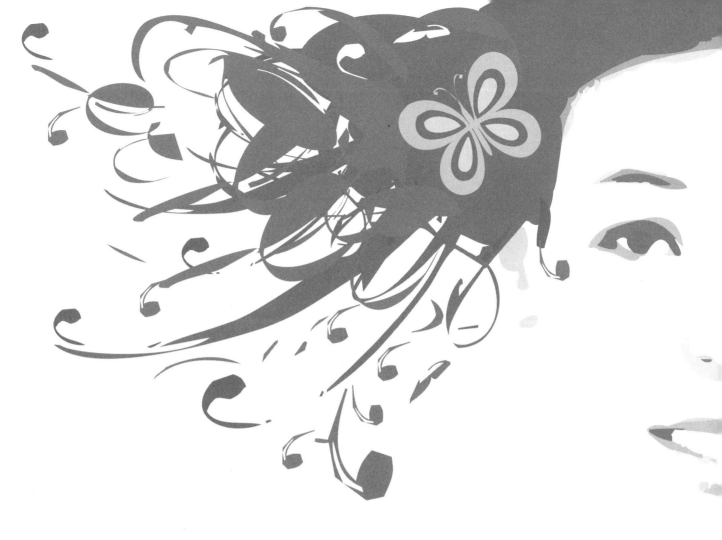

Success Can Be Yours

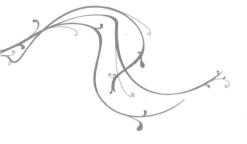

Success Can Be Yours

*You have the power to change
your future – be courageous!*

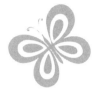

Making your health and your appearance a priority can be challenging, especially if you have many demands on your time and energy.

It's important to devote some time each day to taking care of yourself mentally, emotionally and physically. You will not only look better, but you will feel much better about yourself because you made a commitment and followed through. Your commitment will give you strength to continue to move forward to your goal.

In this section you will review your food journals looking for eating patterns. By analyzing your patterns and recognizing areas for improvement, you will be empowering yourself with the knowledge for change.

You will be introduced to a new recording, *"Imaging Positive Results".* In a state of peaceful relaxation you will be taken through a series of visualizations that will assist you in the positive lifestyle changes you are making. This program is designed to reinforce your desire, determination and motivation toward the achievement of your healthy weight goal. Listen to this

recording as many times as you can while you are progressing through this section. Periodically alternate it with the *"Let's Make an Agreement"* recording.

Rewards are an important part of keeping yourself motivated. Do you ever reward yourself for your accomplishments? You will be making a list of rewards you will give yourself for reaching your intermediate goals. When you make your list, make sure they are rewards that will give you the incentive to reach your goal.

You will also be introduced to setting small goals on a weekly basis. They will help you focus on making small changes in your eating habits.

"Mental Exercise 2" will help you begin to uncover the inner forces that prompt you to overeat. Being truthful as you answer each question may not be easy but it is extremely important to your future success. As you begin to see the relationship between your innermost feelings and experiences and your eating patterns, you will find your relationship with food changing.

A Closer Look at Your Food Journal

It's a good idea to continue to journal your food intake until you complete this program, if not beyond. It will help you stay on track by observing your caloric intake. The longer you keep a food journal, the easier it will get and the more patterns you will see emerging.

In order for you to benefit from recording everything you ate last week, you now need to go back and look at what you ate through different eyes. Analyze each meal as to its nutritional value and calorie content. In a separate notebook make notes of how you could change the meal to be lower in calories and more healthful. As you analyze each meal make some meal plans to follow next week. You could make this a family activity by asking your children to help you plan and prepare healthy meals.

As you review each meal keep in mind the following:

- There is more nutritional value in fresh vegetables than in canned or frozen vegetables.

- High fiber whole wheat or multi-grain bread is more nutritious than white bread.

- Fried foods are higher in calories and more unhealthy than foods that are baked or broiled.

- Snacks comprised of chips and dips contain mostly empty calories (no nutritional value). Substitute fruit or vegetables.

- Most fast foods are higher in calories than those you prepare at home.

It's unreasonable to expect to change everything all at once. We live in a very fast paced, busy society that sometimes makes unreasonable demands on our time and energies. You may already feel you are pushed to your limit juggling your time between your job, your children and their activities, and your household responsibilities. You probably have little, if any, time left over to plan, let alone prepare, nutritious meals. It's much easier to frequent the drive-thru of one of the fast-food establishments or to call your local pizza restaurant that delivers.

You can begin by making small changes. The more changes you make to the healthy side of the ledger the quicker you will reach your goal. You can greatly reduce your calorie intake by eating less fast food meals per week. Replace those meals with foods you prepare yourself, based on healthy food choices. If you have to eat fast food, instead of the cheeseburger, fries and soft drink, order the grilled chicken sandwich and an apple. Better yet, order one of their salads with olive oil and lemon or vinegar.

It's important for you to start reading labels and compare fat, fiber and calorie content and choose the ones lower in calories and sugar content. Try to find food items to substitute whenever possible. For example, substitute high calorie sugar sweetened jams and jellies, with jams and jellies sweetened with fruit juices. Every small step along the way will help you move closer and closer toward your goal!

Knowledge is Power

Devote a few minutes every day to educating yourself on the guidelines for healthy eating and nutrition. You will find some excellent resources on our web site www.bodyesteem.com to get you started.

Goal Setting

At the beginning of every week, set a goal for the week.

Your goals could include:

- Eating smaller portions
- Not eating in front of the TV
- Including more raw vegetables
- Choosing not to drink sodas
- Choosing not to eat fast food

- Choosing not to eat snacks
- Choosing not to eat desserts
- Choosing not to eat candy
- Choosing to eat more meals you have prepared
- Choosing not to eat frozen foods

Write your goal for the week on several 3x5 cards or sticky notes. Place one on your refrigerator and the others where you will see them several times during the day.

Don't think in terms of "I can't ever have _____ for the rest of my life." Rather, say to yourself, "just for today I choose not to have _____. I can have it tomorrow, but just for today I am choosing to eliminate _____."

If you do this every day you will find you are not feeling restricted or deprived, you are willingly making the choices that will change your life in a positive and beneficial way. Remind yourself that you have decided to eat healthier because you will look and feel better. You will soon find your new way of eating is automatic and you'll think of it as your "normal" way of eating.

As you change your eating habits you are developing new patterns you will live with for the rest of your life. Imagine a future where you will feel better, have more energy and never have to "diet" again. Remind yourself daily about why you started this program.

Focus on a slim and healthy future becoming your reality and it will soon be yours.

A New Awareness

As you tune into your body and become aware of your behaviors, you will notice there are "danger" times, i.e. eating when you are not physically hungry, eating out of boredom, when you are depressed, or when you need comforting, etc. It's at these critical moments, you can replace eating with a positive behavior. Add your own positive behaviors to the examples below.

Examples:

- Write some positive things about yourself in a journal.

- Close your eyes and visualize the person you want to become.

- Make a list of the foods you are choosing to say "NO" to.

- Make a shopping list of healthy snacks.

- Listen to one of the recordings in this program.

MY POSITIVE BEHAVIORS

1. _____
2. _____
3. _____
4. _____
5. _____

Incorporate them the next time you feel like eating outside of your normal mealtime schedule.

As you work with this program and begin to uncover the unconscious reasons underlying your overweight, you will find those "danger" times popping up less and less and your need to eat between meals becoming an activity of the past.

Guidelines for Success

You will be faced with many challenges and temptations as you proceed toward the achievement of your weight goal. Following these guidelines will help guarantee your success. You may want to refer to this list weekly to help you stay on track.

Clean Your Closet

As you start to release the pounds and inches your clothes are going to get too big for you. When this happens, clean out your closet. Get rid of your *fat* clothes or find a seamstress or tailor to take them in for you. If you leave them in your closet, you are accepting it's OK for you to gain the weight again - you already have the wardrobe. Why not donate your old clothes to a local charity or thrift store. GAINING WEIGHT SHOULDN'T BE EASY. The harder you make it for yourself, the easier it will be to maintain your losses.

Buy Form Fitting Clothes

Tent dresses or floats make even a slim person look fat. They also allow you to gain a lot of excess pounds without feeling uncomfortable. When you buy new clothes, select clothes that are form fitting and reveal your body. You will be more aware of any changes in your weight, and you can take action before one pound becomes twenty. You will also be more aware of your losses when your zippers zip easier and you move your belt to the next smaller notch. Buy at least one item that is a size smaller than you are wearing so you have a goal to work towards.

Take Pictures of Your Progress

Have someone take a picture of you each time you reach one of your intermediate goals. Don't be surprised if you see a happier, more positive person looking back at you.

Set Reasonable and Realistic Goals

If your goals are unrealistic you are setting yourself up for failure and self-punishment. A reasonable, sustainable weight loss goal is 4-10 pounds per month, but keep in mind, this depends on your body type and lifestyle. You may lose more in the beginning and your weight loss will slow as you get close to your goal.

Don't Skip Meals

Your body is like a machine. It needs fuel to burn fat and run efficiently. The less frequently you eat, the slower your metabolism becomes. As your metabolism slows, your body begins to store fat cells and water for periods of starvation. Eating regularly and drinking water will insure your metabolism is functioning at peak efficiency.

If You Have A Craving, Wait

Wait at least 10 minutes before giving in to your cravings. First, drink some water and then proceed with one of the "positive behaviors" you listed in "A New Awareness" on page 52. You will probably find the craving is gone after this time – but – if it isn't try to find the healthiest substitute possible.

Eat Slowly

Studies have shown it takes approximately twenty minutes for the food that reaches your stomach lining to be broken down so it can be assimilated into your blood stream, for the assimilation to take place, and for your blood to carry the message that nourishment has been received to the hunger centers in your brain. A surprisingly small amount of food is sufficient to trigger the signal.

Some tips to help you slow your pace:
- Listen to mellow music while you are eating.
- Cut your food into small bite-size portions.
- Chew your food slowly, for as long as possible.
- Set your knife and fork down between bites.
- Try eating with the opposite hand.
- TALK, TALK, TALK. It's difficult to talk and eat at the same time.
- Wait to start eating until everyone else has been served.

Eating slowly accomplishes three important things:
- It allows your digestion to be more natural.
- Slowing your pace improves assimilation of nutrients.
- You won't be taking in as many calories in the twenty minute period.

Enjoy Your Food

Enjoying this life means taking time not just to smell the flowers, but also the food you eat. Enjoy the nuances of the aromas released by your meal and savor each bite. Notice the more subtle textures of the food. Consider the differences between raw and cooked veggies. You might be surprised how good healthy eating can help expand your pallet and improve your skills in the kitchen.

Eat Only When You Are Sitting Down

If you make it a rule to sit down and eat you won't be snacking on the run. It also forces you to become more aware of the food you are eating. Choose to eat in only one room, in one particular place. After you sit down, WAIT. Take three or four slow, deep breaths before you begin to eat. This will help you relax and eat more slowly.

Leave Some Food on Your Plate

Overcoming a childhood program that required you to clean your plate because of the poor starving children in "_____" takes a conscious effort on your part. Giving yourself permission to leave food on your plate will help you overcome any guilt feelings you may experience and make you more aware of the portion size that is healthy.

You will need this behavior when eating out where the portions have become too large for one person. What you serve yourself in any situation is only an estimate of what you think it will take to satisfy you - you may have guessed wrong. Look at it this way - the portion of food you leave on your plate just means you will weigh that much less tomorrow.

Tune In To Your Body

Eat slowly, chew your food thoroughly and check in with your body throughout your meal to see how you are feeling. Stop eating for a minute or two and see how you feel. Eat only until you are satisfied and no longer hungry, **not** until you are full. Take small bites and really chew your food to aid in digestion. We have important enzymes that are released in our mouth which begins the digestion process, consider this as you are chewing. Also try to limit your liquid intake while eating.

Eat Foods You Have Prepared

Cooking the foods you eat will encourage food awareness. It requires a lot more effort than stopping at a restaurant where all the work is done for you behind the scenes, but delivers much more than just a meal. It will also make you aware of the amount of sugar and other high calorie ingredients that make up those "goodies" you might find hard to avoid. Taking the time to prepare something will force you to consider what you're putting into your body and offers an excellent opportunity for a chance to create a healthy alternative to the calorie loaded restaurant and frozen foods.

Eat Everything Off A Small Plate

That includes snack food too. Eating potato chips, cookies, nuts, or candies piecemeal, casually, or on the run, can result in consuming amounts that would appall you if they were piled on a single plate.

Plan Your Meals for a Week

Take the time to plan your meals and snacks for a week. The time you spend will pay off when you are shopping and when you are preparing your meals. This is also a good opportunity for you to change your family to a healthier way of eating as well.

Don't Shop On An Empty Stomach

Everything looks and smells good - too good - when you are hungry. You'll be feeling low and the junk food will be twice as hard to pass up. Wait until you have eaten and are calm and in charge of the situation before you fill your shopping cart.

Shop With A List

Make your grocery list based on your meal plans and purchase *only* the items on your list. Avoid impulse purchases of supermarket "specials" and end-of-aisle "sales".

Shop On the Perimeter of the Store

Grocery stores usually keep the healthy food on the perimeter of the store, that's where you'll find all your fresh food. Start first in the produce section and work your way around from there.

Write Your Goals And Inspirations At The Top Of Your Grocery List

This will remind you to buy foods that will keep you on track and help support your healthy lifestyle. For example: "Eat organic produce," "Sugar is the devil," "My body is more important than corporate profits!"

Buy Only Foods That Will Help You Achieve Your Goal

Don't buy foods you have trouble resisting and know are unhealthy for you.

At work, remove food from your immediate work area, including those chocolate cookies in your bottom desk drawer. Put them where they belong - in the lunch room. Better yet, toss them in the garbage. If you have a problem trashing food, make an anonymous community offering in the lunch room. Don't replace them after the masses have feasted on the food that keeps you unhealthy. If food is not readily available, you will not have to use your willpower so often to resist it and you won't feel as deprived.

Discuss Food Only At the Table

Talking about food and diets only makes you more aware of food at the time - and - bores other people.

Avoid "All You Can Eat" Restaurants

Select restaurants that serve the foods you can and should eat. Avoid reading the menu and order only what you know is healthy and nutritious and will further your efforts to reach your weight goal. Order before the others in your party so you will not be tempted to order the foods chosen by others.

Learn About Nutrition

The body you are now inhabiting is the only one you will ever have. Learning and practicing proper nutrition will help you live a longer, healthier, more productive life.

Learn To Recognize Emotional Hunger

Learn to recognize the difference between physical hunger and the emotional urge to eat. Learn to trust your body and its signals. Eat only when you are physically hungry, and eat only enough to satisfy that physical need. Let your body tell you when, what, and how much to eat.

Don't eat when you feel:

Angry	Upset	Sad
Lonely	Depressed	Anxious
Bored	Frustrated	Insecure
Stressed		

Instead of reaching for food - reach for one of the CD's in this program. Each CD contains "less than 0 calories" and will help you deal with the feelings triggering your emotional hunger.

Take It One Day At A Time

Thinking you can *never* have another piece of Cherry Cheesecake or a Hot Fudge Sundae, could be a pretty discouraging thought. Adopt the attitude of "one day at a time" and think, "just for today I will reject the foods I crave. Tomorrow I can have all I want, but just for today I will eat healthy and nutritious foods".

If you repeat that phrase every morning, and when you are faced with a temptation, you will find it easier to resist those foods that have made it necessary for you to be on this program in the first place.

TV and Commercials

When a food commercial comes on TV - WALK, STRETCH, MOVE ABOUT, or CHANGE THE CHANNEL, but don't nibble. Walk anywhere except into the kitchen. As you are moving, think about the powerful ways advertisers manipulate you into desiring completely unhealthy food.

Blowing It

Going off your healthy eating lifestyle or "blowing it" by eating something you think is "bad" shouldn't give you permission to overeat or eat high calorie foods for the rest of the day. And remember – eating something "bad" doesn't make you "bad." Make a list of all of the good things you have done like not having your morning doughnut. Forgive yourself - one piece of chocolate cake didn't make you fat. Get back on track and resolve to do better tomorrow.

Reward Yourself

Be glad you are finally doing something good for yourself and your body. Reward yourself (with something other than food) for reaching your intermediate goals. Be proud of yourself for finally taking the action to become a slimmer, healthier person.

Keep Busy - In Body and Mind

Becoming bored can be dangerous if you are conditioned to eat in response to boredom. If you feel boredom setting in, engage in some form of stimulating activity - call a friend, take a walk, or start a craft project, until the feeling passes.

Develop a Support System

Solicit support from your spouse, family and best friends. Studies show that dieters who are complimented, encouraged and given positive support, lose more weight and maintain better than those who are not encouraged during the tough times.

"No" Yourself

Learn to say NO to that little voice within that tells you the chocolate cake would taste really good right now and would make you feel better. Of course it would taste good – but would it really make you feel better? You'd probably feel guilty and then you'd want to eat more – and then you'd feel even more guilty and . . . ! Remind that little voice that you are in the process of changing your life in a positive way and its support would be nice. The next time that little voice tries to sabotage you – just tell it to "Shut Up." And remember - slim people make choices daily that guarantee they will maintain their ideal weight.

Choose to Eat Healthy

Be aware of the foods you are eating. Are they natural or are they full of additives? Have they been processed in a way that retains the nutritional value or are they nothing but empty calories? Be mindful of the food you are putting in your body.

Rewards for Releasing Weight

Make a list of the rewards you will give yourself for reaching your intermediate goals.

These rewards should be special and meaningful. Do something nice for your body such as a massage at a spa, a new haircut, or a manicure. Or perhaps, you could take a weekend trip or send yourself flowers. Maybe it's a new article of clothing that would give you the incentive you need to really stick to your diet and exercise program.

5# _____	60# _____
10# _____	65# _____
15# _____	70# _____
20# _____	75# _____
25# _____	80# _____
30# _____	85# _____
35# _____	90# _____
40# _____	95# _____
45# _____	100# _____
50# _____	

Cut out pictures from magazines that represent your rewards for losing weight. Paste them on the following pages or on a piece of poster board. Refer to them daily. Be sure to reward yourself when you reach each intermediate goal.

My Rewards

My Rewards

Choose a time and location where you can be undisturbed for at least 20 minutes. If possible have your CD player within easy reach so you can pause it when instructed to do so during the exercise.

Listen to **CD II – Track 3** and mentally ask yourself the following questions when instructed to do so. **Trust the first answer that comes into your mind** and write it in the space provided.

> <u>Note:</u> **If you encounter repressed or forgotten experiences that are upsetting, uncomfortable, or cause you to become very emotional and your emotional stability is being affected, consult a professional counselor who can help you uncover and resolve the experiences you have been repressing.**

Mental Exercise 2

These questions and statements are designed to open up, stimulate, and extend insight into your weight problem. As you read each question, take some time to think about your answer. If you start to feel uncomfortable it's an indication this is a sensitive area and you need to look at it in more depth. Be truthful with yourself, for only in uncovering the inner forces that prompt you to overeat, will you be in a position to change your destructive eating patterns.

When and why did my health and appearance become a lower priority for me? _____

_____

The circumstances in my life at that time were _____

_____

Is there a relationship between the circumstances and my weight gain? YES ___ NO ___
If yes, how do they relate? _____

What purpose is the weight serving for me? _____

Why have I not lost the weight? _____

My reasons now for losing the weight are _____

_____

Are these reasons strong enough to change my eating habits? YES _____ NO _____

Do I really WANT to lose weight? YES ___ NO ___

Do I NEED to lose weight? YES ___ NO ___

Do I HAVE to lose weight? YES ___ NO ___

Am I AFRAID to lose the weight? YES ___ NO ___

Am I COMMITTED to losing weight? YES ___ NO ___

Am I COMMITTED to reaching my goal? YES ___ NO ___

What am I willing to do to reach my weight goal? _____
_____

How much control do I have in releasing the weight? _____
_____

How much responsibility do I have for releasing the weight? _____
_____

Are there any advantages to staying exactly as I am? YES ___ NO ___
If yes, what are they? _____

What are the disadvantages of staying exactly as I am at this time? _____
_____

Do I deserve to be slim? YES ___ NO ___
If, no, why not? _____

Do I have a fear of being slim? YES ___ NO ___

Have I ever been slim for a long period of time? YES ___ NO ___

Did anything catastrophic happen? YES ___ NO ___
If yes, what? _____

Was it really so bad? YES ___ NO ___

How is that experience affecting my weight now? _____
_____

What would I have to do to put the negative part of that experience behind me and move on? _____
_____

If I were slim, how would my life change? _____
_____

Could I live with the changes? YES ___ NO ___

Is it possible for me to be slim without changing anything else in my life? YES ___ NO ___
If no, what would have to change? _____

How are my sex drive and my sexual responses being affected by my being overweight? _____
_____

Am I afraid of the changes that may take place in my sex drive and my sexual responses when I am at my ideal weight? YES ___ NO ___
If YES, why? _____

When was the last time I **REALLY** looked at myself in a full-length mirror? _____

Did I like what I saw? YES ___ NO ___

If I had a magic wand and could change my appearance, what would I change and how would I look?
_____

Is there anything or anyone stopping me from making those changes now? YES ___ NO ___
If yes, what would I have to do to overcome the obstacles that stand in my way of making the changes?
_____

Is there anyone in my life who will not support me in my commitment to changing my life in this positive way? YES ___ NO ___

If yes, who and why would they not want me to be successful? _____

_____

If YES, can I be successful without their support?   YES ___ NO ___

If NO, what can I do to gain their support and encouragement? _____

_____

 Turn your CD player back on and relax as you listen to the suggestions that will assist you in reaching your weight goal.

You have the power and ability to achieve and maintain your ideal weight. The more you believe in yourself the easier it will be to overcome any obstacles on your path to achieving your goal!

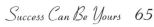

Wrap-Up

CONGRATULATIONS – YOU HAVE COMPLETED "SUCCESS CAN BE YOURS."

As you continue on your journey, this is where you weigh and measure yourself and chart your progress. Know that there are changes taking place at deeper levels of your consciousness that will begin to manifest on the physical level as you proceed through the program. The more involved you are, the more apparent those changes will be.

Reading your "*Weight Loss Agreement*" every day before breakfast will reinforce your desire, determination and commitment to accomplishing your goal. If your motivation weakens, listen to the "*Let's Make an Agreement*" recording when you go to sleep at night to increase your motivation. As you begin to see and feel the results of your efforts, your determination and commitment to reaching your goal will increase.

As you know, your weight is determined by the number of calories you eat each day minus what your body uses. Regular physical activity uses the extra calories that would otherwise be stored as fat. When you combine daily exercise along with cutting your calorie intake you will lose weight more quickly than dieting or exercise alone. Wouldn't you agree that "diet" and "exercise" are the ideal couple to include on your Body Esteem journey?

Setting and accomplishing weekly goals is another way to stay committed and involved with the program and you also get to reward yourself on a weekly basis when you accomplish those goals. Additionally, you get to feel good because you followed through. It's a WIN WIN WIN situation. Writing your weekly goal at the top of your grocery list and on a 3x5 card you place on your refrigerator will help insure you reach your goals.

Re-doing those pesky food journals is a great way to get your family involved in healthier eating. It can be an educational experience for the whole family that could result in longer, healthier lives for everyone.

The "*Guidelines for Success*" will help you stay on track as you progress on your journey. Incorporate a few of the ones you think are most important now, if you haven't already, and add several new ones on a weekly basis. They are all worthy of your attention.

What did you choose for your rewards? A day at the spa, flowers, a new piece of jewelry, a manicure and/or pedicure, a facial, a full body massage, a new dress, a purse or pair of shoes, a makeover at your favorite salon? Whatever will motivate you to reach your goals – you go for it girl!

"*Mental Exercise 2*" was designed to help you begin to uncover and resolve the inner forces that prompt you to overeat. Repeating this exercise more than once will allow you to discover additional roadblocks to your success. Aren't you curious about what else might be lurking under the surface of your consciousness?

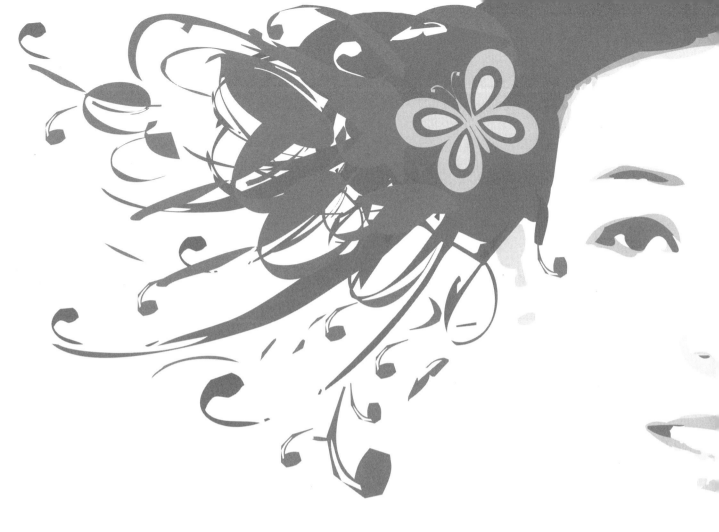

Self Evaluation

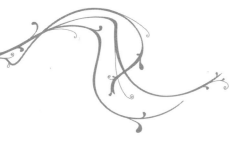

Self Evaluation

Discovery is the path to change!

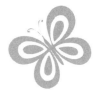

Are you ready to make some exciting discoveries? In this section you will be looking at your attitudes toward weight and analyzing the answers. Allow yourself to take a step back and see yourself from a different perspective.

"Mental Exercise 3" will help you begin to discover the deeper reasons behind your overweight. Trust the first answer that comes into your mind and write it down. Don't try to analyze it at that point, just continue answering the questions. You can go back and look at them in more depth later.

Remember, the more open you are, the more successful you will be in receiving the answers that will allow you to reach your goals.

How do you respond to food? Becoming aware of your responses will help you change them.

Is your perception of yourself accurate? We seldom see ourselves as others see us. The written exercises in this section will help you discover if you have been discounting or ignoring the positive aspects of who you really are. Adjusting your vision to see yourself as a beautiful woman, might take some time, but it's an important step to discovering your true Body Esteem.

In the *"Self Talk"* exercise you will make a list of the negative things you tell yourself about your appearance and you will then re-program yourself with positive statements. After all, isn't it time to let go of all the negative self-judgement you've been carrying and start to really enjoy this life?

Listen to the *"Imaging Positive Results"* recording on a daily basis. Continue to read your *"Weight Loss Agreement"* every morning and listen to the *"Let's Make an Agreement"* recording at least once. You may also listen to either recording as you go to sleep at night.

Attitudes About Weight

Circle or highlight the underlined word, or words, that best completes each sentence. Once again, take some time to think about your answers. Think about how you feel about other overweight people you know and how you REALLY feel about yourself.

Slim people are <u>weak</u>, <u>strong</u>, <u>overbearing</u>, <u>vulnerable</u>.

<u>Slim</u>, <u>overweight</u> people have more fun.

Obesity is a <u>physical</u>, <u>mental</u>, <u>emotional</u> problem.

I will be <u>more</u>, <u>less</u> attractive at my desired weight.

I will love myself <u>more</u>, <u>less</u>, <u>the same</u> when I reach my weight goal.

My family will love me <u>more</u>, <u>less</u>, <u>the same</u> when I reach my weight goal.

When I look at myself in a mirror I feel <u>good</u>, <u>bad</u>, <u>indifferent</u> about what I see.

Overweight people are <u>more</u>, <u>less</u>, <u>equally</u> as lovable as slim people.

I <u>am</u>, <u>am not</u> lovable.

I <u>am</u>, <u>am not</u> motivated to release my excess weight.

I <u>am</u>, <u>am not</u> committed to releasing my excess weight. % of commitment _____

I <u>do</u>, <u>do not</u> have control over my weight.

I <u>do</u>, <u>do not</u> respond to temptations by eating.

I <u>do</u>, <u>do not</u> respond to frustrations by eating.

I <u>do</u>, <u>do not</u> respond to conflicts by eating.

I <u>do</u>, <u>do not</u> respond to anxiety by eating.

I <u>do</u>, <u>do not</u> respond to rejection by eating.

I <u>do</u>, <u>do not</u> respond to stressful situations by eating.

I <u>do</u>, <u>do not</u> solve my problems by eating.

I <u>can</u>, <u>can not</u> live with sustained thinness.

NOW: Read over your answers as if another person had written them.
What do they tell you about that person and their attitudes about weight?
What advice would you give someone with these responses about releasing their weight?
Can you follow your own advice?   YES ___   NO ___

Choose a time and location where you can be undisturbed for at least 20 minutes. If possible have your CD player within easy reach so you can pause it when instructed to do so during the exercise.

Listen to **CD II – Track 3** and mentally ask yourself the following questions when instructed to do so. **Trust the first answer that comes into your mind** and write it in the space provided.

> <u>Note:</u> **If you encounter repressed or forgotten experiences that are upsetting, uncomfortable, or cause you to become very emotional and your emotional stability is being affected, consult a professional counselor who can help you uncover and resolve the experiences you have been repressing.**

Mental Exercise 3

These questions are designed to help you discover the deeper reasons behind your overweight. As you read each question listen to your inner voice (that little voice inside of you that sometimes sounds like your conscience) for an answer to the question. The more open you are, the more successful you will be in receiving the answers that will allow you to free yourself from your weight prison. Don't rush - take plenty of time with each question, as you need to allow time for the information to filter up to your conscious awareness.

What is my benefit (payoff) for being overweight and living an unhealthy lifestyle? _____

_____

Who is supporting and encouraging me to be overweight? _____

What **foods** are contributing to my being overweight? _____

_____

What suppressed **emotions** are contributing to my unhealthy lifestyle? _____

_____

What am I telling other people about myself by being overweight? _____

_____

How do I REALLY feel about myself? _____

_____

Is there an experience I am suppressing from my consciousness that is contributing to my being overweight?
YES ___ NO ___

If YES, am I emotionally ready to deal with the memories of that experience at my conscious level of awareness? YES ___ NO ___

If YES, what is the next step I need to take to free myself from the effects that experience has had on the way I relate to food and my health? _____

Is there more than one experience I am suppressing from my consciousness that is contributing to my being overweight? YES ___ NO ___

Where will I be one year from now if I proceed on my present unhealthy course? _____

_____

Turn your CD player back on and relax as you listen to the suggestions that will assist you in reaching your weight goal.

Food Responsiveness -1

Check the answer that best completes the statement.

I think I am a compulsive eater.   YES ___   NO ___

I often eat when I am not really hungry.   YES ___   NO ___   SOMETIMES ___

I feel guilty after I overeat.   YES ___   NO ___   SOMETIMES ___

I feel guilty if I skip a meal.   YES ___   NO ___   SOMETIMES ___

Check all statements that apply to you:

Thinking about my favorite food . . .

___   Causes me to feel hungry
___   Makes my mouth water
___   Causes me to go to the refrigerator to get something to eat
___   Has no effect upon me

Seeing food . . .

___   Causes me to feel hungry
___   Makes my mouth water
___   Causes me to go to the refrigerator to get something to eat
___   Has no effect upon me

Smelling food . . .

___   Causes me to feel hungry
___   Makes my mouth water
___   Causes me to go to the refrigerator to get something to eat
___   Has no effect upon me

Watching others eat . . .

___   Causes me to feel hungry
___   Makes my mouth water
___   Causes me to go to the refrigerator to get something to eat
___   Has no effect upon me
___   Causes me to want to eat too

I respond to food commercials on television by . . .

____ Going to the refrigerator to get something to eat
____ Turning them off
____ Buying the food they are advertising
____ Ignoring them

If I take a bite of cake, cookie, ice cream or candy . . .

____ I can't stop until I have eaten it all
____ I am able to take one bite and stop
____ I make up excuses so I won't feel guilty for eating it all
____ I am unaware that I am eating it all until it is gone

I experience cravings for food . . .

____ When I first wake up
____ 1 Hour after waking up
____ Within 30 minutes after eating a meal
____ Just before bedtime
____ When I watch television
____ When I am lonely
____ When I am depressed
____ When the weather is dreary
____ Never

I think about food . . .

____ When I am planning a meal
____ When I am preparing a meal
____ When I am eating a meal
____ All the time

The last time I said "NO" to a high calorie dessert was _____

I made healthy choices _____ times in the last week

Check the statement which best describes how you feel about food . . .

____ I eat to live
____ I live to eat

You can completely eliminate cigarettes from your life –

you can completely eliminate alcohol from your life –

you can completely eliminate drugs from your life –

but you cannot completely eliminate food from your life.

Eating Patterns

The physical sensations I experience when my body is telling me it is in need of food are:

1. _____
2. _____
3. _____
4. _____
5. _____

The physical sensations I experience when my emotions are prompting me to eat are:

1. _____
2. _____
3. _____
4. _____
5. _____

I feel sleepy or lethargic after eating the following foods:

1. _____
2. _____
3. _____
4. _____
5. _____

I feel energized after eating the following foods:

1. _____
2. _____
3. _____
4. _____
5. _____

Caffeine causes me to feel...

_____ Jittery
_____ Alert
_____ Has no effect on my system

I often crave...

_____ Sweets   _____ Fried Foods
_____ Meat   _____ Spicy Foods
_____ Potatoes   _____ Snack Foods
_____ Pasta

The foods I normally crave when I am on a diet are:

1. _____
2. _____
3. _____
4. _____
5. _____

In order of seriousness, my poor eating habits are:

1. _____
2. _____
3. _____
4. _____
5. _____

Taking each of my poor eating habits in order, I could change each habit into a positive action to support and assist me in reaching my goals by:

1. _____
2. _____
3. _____
4. _____
5. _____

I use food for _____

Eating food sometimes satisfies my emotional need for _____

I would satisfy these needs if food was not available by _____

As a child my snacks usually consisted of _____

My snacks now consist of _____

The foods I regularly eat that I know are high in calories, low in nutritional value and have caused me to gain weight are:

1. _____
2. _____
3. _____
4. _____
5. _____

The foods I know to be healthy and nutritious, low in calories, and will assist me in obtaining my weight goals are:

1. _____
2. _____
3. _____
4. _____
5. _____

The foods I now CHOOSE to eliminate from my nutritional program are:

1. _____
2. _____
3. _____
4. _____
5. _____

The foods I now CHOOSE to eat are:

1. _____
2. _____
3. _____
4. _____
5. _____

In the presence of food, ask yourself -
How much do I WANT?
How much do I really NEED?

Self Perception

When you look in a mirror, is the reflection you see looking back at you the real you, or only a representation of how you think and feel about yourself? Does a good or bad hair day affect the way you feel? Have you ever been surprised by comments that others have made to you about how you look?

We seldom see ourselves
as others see us

If you are sensitive about your weight and your appearance, some of these questions may be difficult for you to answer. If you can, it will be to your benefit to push yourself a little bit and go beyond your comfort zone, for only in doing so will you be able to change the patterns and behaviors that have resulted in your being overweight.

Look in a full-length mirror. Write a detailed physical description of the person you see in the mirror. (Be sure to include your positive attributes as well as what you consider to be your negatives.)

_____

_____

_____

_____

Write a detailed description of how you think other people see you.

_____

_____

_____

_____

Does the person you see in the mirror match the description of how you think other people see you?
YES ___ NO ___

If they are different, how are they different? _____

_____

Write a detailed description of how you think your family sees you. _____

_____

_____

_____

Does the person you see in the mirror match the description of how you think your family sees you?
YES ___ NO ___

If they are different, how are they different? _____

_____

Do you think your family sees you the same way others see you?   YES ___ NO ___

If no, why do you think your family sees you differently? _____

_____

If it's not too embarrassing, ask a friend and a family member to write detailed descriptions of how they see you. Ask them to be honest. Compare their descriptions with the ones you wrote.

How does your friend's description differ from your description? _____

_____

How does your family's description differ from your description? _____

_____

Why do you think they are different? _____

_____

Which description do you think is the real you?

_____ The reflection you see in the mirror

_____ The description of how you think other people see you

_____ The description of how you think your family sees you

_____ The description written by a friend

_____ The description written by your family

_____ None of the above

Write a description of how you would like to be and how you would like other people to perceive you. This could be a description of how you would like to be in the future. _____

_____

_____

_____

Remember: Be as honest with yourself as you can, for only by being honest will you begin to open yourself to making the changes that will allow you to become the person you would like to be. Have you considered that by not being honest with yourself, you may be discounting or ignoring all of the positive aspects of who you really are?

Go back and re-read the answers you just wrote and ask yourself if you are really being honest with yourself If you can honestly answer YES, then you are done with this exercise.

If you have any doubts, or if your answer is a definite NO, there is a part of you that does not want you to change. Challenge that part of you that wants to remain in control and re-write any answers where you feel you were being less than honest.

Change is usually not easy or comfortable, but it is rewarding. As you allow yourself to take those steps that will change your future, realize you will soon become comfortable with the new you and if you were to return to the way you are now it would be uncomfortable and unacceptable.

Be strong and move forward with courage and conviction. It won't be easy and there will be times when you just want to say "forget this," but remember, each positive step you take is moving you closer to the future you desire.

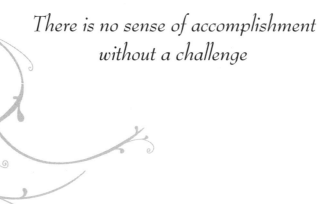

*There is no sense of accomplishment
without a challenge*

Self Talk

Do you know your thinking is the greatest factor in influencing your appearance and estimation of yourself? In other words, you are what you think you are. The way you look today is the result of how you feel about yourself and the negative or positive way you have been programming yourself. Your thoughts and feelings about yourself are simply a matter of conditioning and may go as far back as your childhood and you can change them.

A negative thought is just as effective as a positive one. Every time you have a negative thought about yourself and your appearance you are reinforcing it. How long have you been unhappy with the way you look? How many times a day do you think or say "I'm too fat?" Probably a lot! How many times a day do you say "I am slender and healthy?" Probably never!

Now is the appropriate time for you to re-program your thinking in a positive way.

Make a list of all the **negative** things you have been telling yourself about your appearance.

Example: "I'm fat."

1. _____
2. _____
3. _____
4. _____
5. _____

Now, write each negative as a **positive statement** that supports the way you want to look after you have reached your goal. Write it as if it was an already accomplished fact.

Example: "I am slender and healthy."

1. _____
2. _____
3. _____
4. _____
5. _____

Make several copies of the list of positive statements you just wrote. Put a copy on your refrigerator and several other places where you will see it frequently. Repeat your new positive statements every time you see the list.

As you repeat your new positive statements, your thinking will change. The more you repeat these statements, the faster your thinking will change. As your thinking changes, your body will change to reflect your new positive attitude about yourself and your appearance.

Wrap-Up

CONGRATULATIONS – YOU HAVE COMPLETED "SELF EVALUATION." Weigh yourself and chart your progress. Reward yourself (with something other than food) – YOU DESERVE IT.

There were lots of opportunities in this section to make some exciting discoveries about yourself and your feelings about being overweight. Remember as you work with each exercise, there are no right or wrong answers. There are only your answers and how they relate to you. As you look at each question, you might repeat it in your mind several times and then wait for the answer. Trust the first answer that comes into your mind and write it down.

Are you having difficulty looking at your attitudes about weight and what triggers you to eat when you're not really hungry? Close your eyes and ask yourself why you are having difficulty answering these questions. Sit quietly for a minute or two and become aware of anything you see, feel or hear that could explain your reluctance to uncovering the truth.

It's ok for you to go back and re-do any of the exercises if you feel there is still more information for you to discover. It's like peeling the leaves off an artichoke to get to the heart – you have to go through layers of protective consciousness to get to the real reason underlying your weight problem.

"Food Responsiveness" – Make a list of the things that cause you to want to eat. Put the list on your refrigerator door to remind you when you are responding to an outside stimulus rather than a physical need for food.

"Eating Patterns" – Go back and re-read your answers and place a check mark next to the most important things that you want to remember when you are feeling hungry, shopping and preparing meals. Make notes on a 3x5 card that you can carry with you to remind you of the changes you want to make. Refer to them frequently until you have changed your eating patterns.

"Self Perception" – How accurate is your perception of your appearance? We all have a tendency to be too hard on ourselves, playing up what we perceive as our negative attributes and down playing or ignoring our positive characteristics. Begin right now to focus on your positives, build yourself up, congratulate yourself for even the smallest positive changes, become your own cheering section. Start looking at yourself through more positive eyes and you'll be amazed at how quickly you will see yourself changing.

"Self Talk" – Every time you have a negative thought about yourself, you are reinforcing it. Changing your thinking about yourself may not be easy, particularly if focusing on the negatives has been a life long habit. Making the change into becoming a positive thinker and doer will take time, but it is totally worth the effort. Every time you start to say or think something negative about yourself, STOP, and immediately change it into a positive statement. Example: When you start to think "I can't change," stop yourself and change it to "I am changing my life in positive ways." Repeat the positive statement several times, with conviction. The more positive you think and act, the more you will see and attract positive things into your life.

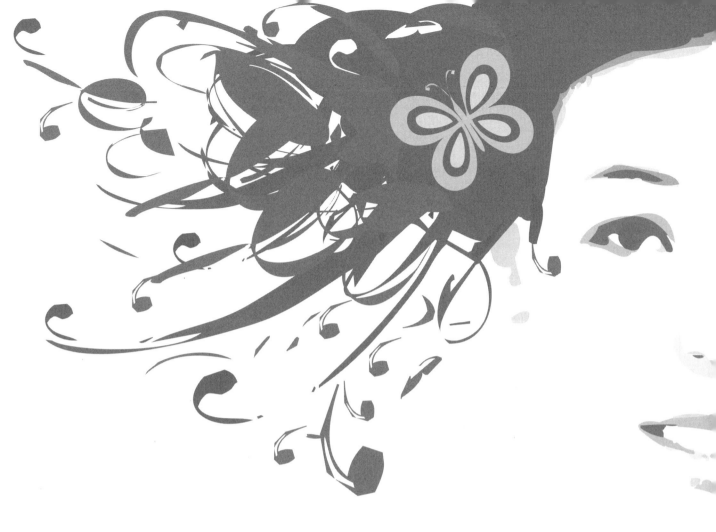

Taking Action

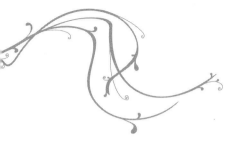

Taking Action

Today is the day!

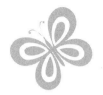

Up to this point the focus of the program has been to make you more aware of your eating patterns and how you respond to food. Hopefully you are thinking more about the nutritional value of the food you eat and making healthier choices.

In this section you're going to begin to focus on your emotions and their relationship to your physical and mental well-being. No aspect of your mental health is more important to the quality and meaning of your existence than emotions. They are what makes your life worth living or they can cause you to feel you have nothing to live for.

Are you aware of how your body responds to the way you think, feel and act? When you are stressed, anxious or angry, your body tries to tell you that something isn't right. You may experience headaches, high blood pressure, neck or back pain, weight gain, and other adverse effects. Your immune system can also be weakened, making you more likely to get colds and other infections.

The reading and written exercises in this section will help you become more familiar with your emotions and the role they play in your health and your interactions with other people.

Just discovering which emotions you are ignoring is only half of the solution – you also need to release your negative emotions. The *"Set Yourself Free"* recording was designed to help you do just that. Through the use of guided imagery you will release the negative emotions you discover. As you do, you will begin to feel lighter and freer, calmer and more at peace.

You will also be introduced to a simple tool that can change your life forever. We all use this tool intentionally or unintentionally. You have either used it to your advantage or it has been a negative influence in your life. This simple tool is Affirmations.

Affirmations are not new. They have been used since humans have had language and can be used to successfully change almost any area of your life. You will create your own personal weight loss affirmation and you will discover a part of you that will try to discourage you from believing you can reach your goal. Through the use of your own personal affirmation, you will effectively reprogram your mind and body to accomplish the positive changes you desire.

Now it's time to take action.

Your Emotions and Your Health

You were born with the capacity to feel and express your emotions. As a baby your only way of communicating your needs to your parents was to cry to get their attention. Before you learned to communicate verbally you may have cried, yelled, screamed or stomped your feet to express your feeling of sadness, anger and frustration.

As you grew older and learned how to tell your parents what you were feeling, you may have been taught it was inappropriate to express your feelings and emotions with words and actions. You may have learned through observation or negative consequences to hide and suppress them.

Unfortunately, the energy it takes to suppress such emotions succeeds in suppressing not only the negative emotions, but other more positive ones as well. Left unexpressed, these emotions can impact your health as well as your behavior. The stress of suppressing these emotions taxes your body's energy and too much stress over a period of time combined with poor coping habits may cause physical, chemical, and hormonal imbalances in the body, which can compromise your health.

A growing body of literature has shown positive and negative emotion-related attitudes and states to be associated with physical and mental health and longevity. Emotion researchers have identified basic emotions such as happiness, sadness, anger, fear, and disgust with differentially patterned autonomic nervous system responses. The healing effect of positive emotions has the potential to reduce stress on your cardiovascular system even in the face of negative life events.

When you don't allow your emotions to flow freely, your body begins to display adverse physical symptoms. Holding in emotion is like compressing a spring. Each time the spring is compressed without releasing it, it builds up more tension or what could be called latent energy. The same principle applies to your feelings and emotions. Take anger for example; the more you suppress your anger or deny it, the tighter that "spring" of anger becomes inside of you, which only gives the anger more power. This latent energy that builds up in your system can eventually get to a point where it causes your body to break down, leading to illness and physical symptoms. This energy of anger may leak out in other ways, such as being overly critical of others and defensive. It can eventually cause you to blow an emotional gasket and fly into fits of rage and even violence.

Dan Winter, a Psychophysiologist, has mapped emotions in the heart and has shown how coherent emotions such as love and appreciation affect the braiding of DNA.

Other researchers have shown coherent emotions produce a heart wave pattern that is smooth and symmetrical; non-coherent emotions (anger, frustration, resentment) produce a jagged wave pattern. Coherent emotions produce heart rate variability, vital for life and health, whereas the negative emotions close the heart down and cause constriction.

Non-coherent emotions also cause suppression of the immune system, hormonal imbalances, inability to think clearly, cardiovascular strain, tumor growth and a negative impact on DNA.

Dr. John Denoliet, University of Antwerp, Belgium, led a study which followed 303 heart patients for six to ten years. He found those hiding negative emotions were four times more likely to die of a heart attack. A similar study conducted by Darla Vale of Rush-Presbyterian-St. Luke Medical Center in Chicago followed 260 women. Those who had heart problems were more anxious and more likely to be suppressing anger.

If you are silently harboring a volcano of negative feelings and emotions, you are greatly increasing your chances of a lethal heart attack as well as impacting your immune system and setting yourself up for other negative health effects.

Get Emotionally Intelligent

When you repeatedly deny a feeling or emotion because you think it is not acceptable you create resistance and stress and tension in your body. It's important for you to learn to accept the feeling or emotion and allow yourself to express it appropriately. It doesn't matter whether it's the reaction to a pleasurable or painful experience, each serves a purpose to your body and learning to accept and release them brings a feeling of peace or relief, returning the body to a state of equilibrium.

If you're thinking the only way to release your feelings and emotions is to verbalize them and that would be too embarrassing or painful . . . I have good news for you. Buy yourself a journal and start writing. Recording your feelings on paper can give you similar feelings of relief and when you go back and read what you have written later, you will see how far you have progressed.

By being able to express and appraise your emotions clearly, understand them, and effectively regulate them, you will experience improved health and well-being. A key to Body Esteem is learning the techniques to acquire and use emotional intelligence. Continue to strive for honesty with yourself and do your best to complete the mental and written exercises in this workbook and you will raise your emotional intelligence and enjoy a brighter future.

Choose a time and location where you can be undisturbed for at least 20 minutes. If possible have your CD player within easy reach so you can pause it when instructed to do so during the exercise.

Listen to **CD II – Track 3** and mentally ask yourself the following questions when instructed to do so. **Trust the first answer that comes into your mind** and write it in the space provided.

> <u>Note:</u> **If you encounter repressed or forgotten experiences that are upsetting, uncomfortable, or cause you to become very emotional and your emotional stability is being affected, consult a professional counselor who can help you uncover and resolve the experiences you have been repressing.**

Mental Exercise 4

All of your emotions, both positive and negative, have an impact on your health and your outlook on life. Expressing your feelings and emotions in a positive way will improve your physical health and metal clarity, and will lead to more satisfying personal relationships.

Negative emotions are heavy emotions. They can weigh you down and hold you back from reaching your full potential, in all areas of your life. These negative emotions have kept your true beauty from manifesting. You can learn to acknowledge and release them before they manifest in excess weight or serious physical problems.

The following questions are designed to help you gain access to the suppressed emotions that could be contributing to your overweight. Read the question, close your eyes and listen for your inner voice to give you the answer. Become aware of anything you hear, feel, or see in your minds eye that represents an answer to the question. Open your eyes and read the question again. When you finish answering the question, close yours eyes and ask yourself: Is the answer related to the cause and the source of my weight problem? Make note of your response. These questions are important, so don't rush your answers. Take plenty of time to get an answer before you move to the next question.

I am angry at myself for _____

_____

I am angry at _____ for _____

I am angry at _____ for _____

I feel guilty about _____

I hate myself for _____

I feel shame about _____

I am afraid of _____

I feel resentful about _____ because
_____

Am I using food in an attempt to suppress my emotions?   YES ___   NO ___
If YES, what emotions have I been "stuffing down" or trying to cover up with food? _____
_____

What physical symptoms do I have that could be a result of withholding these emotions? _____
_____

What are the BEST things that could happen if I stopped suppressing and internalizing these emotions? _____
_____
_____

Who is supporting and encouraging my unhealthy lifestyle? _____
_____

What **foods** are contributing to my being overweight? _____
_____

What suppressed **emotions** are contributing to my unhealthy lifestyle? _____
_____

Turn your CD player back on and relax as you listen to the
suggestions that will assist you in reaching your weight goal.

Suppressed Anger

As a child, were you taught anger was an inappropriate emotion and should be suppressed? Suppressing your anger means it stays bottled up inside and can lead to overeating in an attempt to "stuff it down" or contain it.

Make a list of the people and situations that arouse feelings of anger within you that you may not have expressed.

1. _____
2. _____
3. _____
4. _____
5. _____

Make a list of the things you are angry at yourself about.

1. _____
2. _____
3. _____
4. _____
5. _____

Choose a time and location where you can be undisturbed for at least 20 minutes.

Listen to **CD I – Track 3** and set yourself free.

Note: If you encounter repressed or forgotten experiences that are upsetting, uncomfortable, or cause you to become very emotional and your emotional stability is being affected, consult a professional counselor who can help you uncover and resolve the experiences you have been repressing.

Note: The "*Set Yourself Free*" recording is designed to help you release the negative emotions you listed in "*Mental Exercise 4*" and the "*Suppressed Anger*" exercise. The process that is introduced on this recording may be new to you, but nevertheless, it is very powerful and very effective for releasing even deeply suppressed emotions. Remember, visualizing in your mind's eye is very different than seeing through your physical eyes. Experience it as you did in the test when you recalled and imagined details of your kitchen in your mind. If you are still having difficulty, **pretend** that you are doing it as I describe it. Don't be overly concerned with how you process the information, only that you are able to experience it in some way. Everyone is different and there is no right or wrong way to do it. Be open to the process and create the experience in your own unique way. Continue to work with the recording until you feel you have released all of your suppressed emotions and you are free to move forward with your life in a more positive way. Listen to it periodically to insure that you no longer are being influenced by the "weight" of suppressed negative emotions.

No feeling, no matter how destructive or
disturbing, should ever be suppressed

Affirmations

Before you can expect to change your body you must change the way you think. One of the easiest ways to change your thought patterns is by the use of affirmations. When you affirm something you are making a strong statement that the result you desire is an already accomplished fact. What you are doing is deliberately giving your mind an idea on which to act. It becomes more effective through repetition over a period of time.

Unfortunately, your mind doesn't evaluate whether it's in your best interest. It simply accepts that it is what you want and begins to make the changes necessary to make it your reality. How many times a day do you have negative thoughts about the way you look or feel? How do you think those thoughts have influenced your behavior and your appearance.

Through the use of affirmations you can effectively reprogram your mind and body to accomplish the positive changes you desire. You are already good at the technique, all you have to do is reprogram your thought patterns in a positive way.

Choose one of the affirmations listed on the next page to be your personal weight loss affirmation. Choose one that feels totally right for you. As you begin to repeat it you may feel some emotional resistance at first, especially if it is in strong contrast to the way you have been thinking. The resistance is just that part of you resisting change and growth, and it offers you an opportunity to see what stands between you and your goal.

The more you repeat your affirmation,
the more automatic your responses become.

Repeat your affirmation with strong emotion and firm conviction, with the understanding that as you do you are creating the reality you are stating. By repetition, your mind will begin to believe and then act, without judgment, on the command you are giving it. The more often you say your affirmation the faster it will become a part of your natural thought processes.

Utilize memory joggers as reminders to repeat your affirmation. A memory jogger can be a colored sticker or star attached to your bathroom mirror, refrigerator, steering wheel, telephone, wallet, or any other place you see or use frequently during the day. Each time you see it, mentally repeat your affirmation. Say it to yourself when you are eating, putting on your makeup, taking a shower, stopped at a signal light, or whenever you think of food.

Choose one of the affirmations listed below to be your personal weight loss affirmation.

- I have the power and ability to control my weight
- I easily attain and maintain my ideal weight
- I deserve to be slender and healthy
- Everything I eat turns to health and vitality
- I have the discipline to become thinner and thinner
- I release my emotions in a positive way
- I choose to be free of feeling deprived
- I know what is good for me at all times
- I love myself unconditionally
- I am eating less and enjoying it more
- It's O.K. for me to leave food on my plate
- Everything I eat makes me slimmer and healthier now

My personal affirmation is: _____

_____

Add your personal affirmation on the line below.*

Affirmation

I AM RELEASING THE CONDITIONS OF THE PAST
THAT HAVE CAUSED ME TO BE OVERWEIGHT.

* _____

_____

A SLIM HEALTHY BODY IS MY REALITY.

Look in a mirror and repeat the complete affirmation. Repeat this affirmation many times during the day.

Affirmation Response Exercise

Your mind learns information significantly faster if the statements are written. Write the affirmation that you have chosen to be your personal weight loss affirmation. Next to it write your negative responses or denials to it. Your denial is the little voice inside your head that contradicts the positive things you want to do. In this case it will try to discourage you by giving you negative feedback. Initially write your affirmation twenty to thirty times.

Continue to write your personal affirmation and negative responses at least **ten to fifteen times each day** until you complete this section. Then continue to write your affirmation **ten times a day** until the responses are in agreement with the results you desire to achieve. When your negative feedback becomes a positive response, continue to write only the affirmation, **five times a day** for another ten days. Periodically check your responses to make sure they are still positive. If they become negative, go back to writing the affirmation and responses until your responses become positive again. This may seem tedious, but the results will be worth it.

Affirmation Example	*Response Example*
I have the power and ability to control my weight	Who are you kidding
I have the power and ability to control my weight	Oh yeah, since when
I have the power and ability to control my weight	You never have before, so why now?
I have the power and ability to control my weight	Yeah, right
I have the power and ability to control my weight	Says who
I have the power and ability to control my weight	Ok, maybe you do
I have the power and ability to control my weight	So try it, what have you got to lose
I have the power and ability to control my weight	Yeah, maybe I **can** do it
I have the power and ability to control my weight	I **can** do it
I have the power and ability to control my weight	**I am in control**

Choose a time and location where you can be undisturbed for at least 20 minutes. If possible have your CD player within easy reach so you can pause it when instructed to do so during the exercise.

Listen to **CD II – Track 3** and mentally ask yourself the following questions when instructed to do so. **Trust the first answer that comes into your mind** and write it in the space provided.

> <u>Note:</u> **If you encounter repressed or forgotten experiences that are upsetting, uncomfortable, or cause you to become very emotional and your emotional stability is being affected, consult a professional counselor who can help you uncover and resolve the experiences you have been repressing.**

Mental Exercise 5

The more open you are to the following process, the more successful you will be in receiving the answers that will allow you to free yourself from your weight prison.

As you read each question, if you start to feel nervous or apprehensive it could be an indication the question is significant to your problem. Read the question and then close your eyes and listen to your inner voice for an answer to the question. Anything you hear, feel, or see in your minds eye could be an answer. Don't rush - take plenty of time with each question, as you need to allow time for the information to filter up to your conscious awareness. Record your answer and move on to the next question.

Is there an experience I **am** aware of at my conscious level of awareness that is contributing to my overweight problem?   YES ___   NO ___

If YES, what happened? _____

_____

How old was I? _____ Was anyone else involved?   YES ___   NO ___

If YES, who? _____

When and where did it happen? _____

Did it happen more than once?   YES ___   NO ___

Did I tell anyone about that experience?   YES ___   NO ___

If NO, why not? _____

If YES, who? _____

What was their reaction? _____
_____

Are you angry at the other person involved? YES ___ NO ___

If yes, what would be the worst part of letting the anger go? _____
_____

How or why is that experience preventing me from losing weight? _____
_____

What do I need to do to release myself from the effects of that experience and move on? _____
_____
_____

Besides my weight, what other areas of my life are being affected by that experience? _____
_____

Is there **another experience** I **am** aware of at my conscious level of awareness that is contributing to my overweight problem? YES ___ NO ___

How old was I? _____ Was anyone else involved? YES ___ NO ___

If YES, who? _____

When and where did it happen? _____
_____

Did it happen more than once? YES ___ NO ___

Did I tell anyone about that experience? YES ___ NO ___
If NO, why not? _____

Has that experience affected how I relate to the opposite sex? YES ___ NO ___
If YES, how? _____

Has that experience affected how **I feel about myself**? YES ___ NO ___

If YES, how? _____

What do I need to do to release the effects of that experience and move on with my life? _____
_____

Besides my weight, what other areas of my life are being affected by that experience? _____
_____

What are the best things that could happen if I stop suppressing and internalizing that experience? _____
_____
_____

Is there an experience I **am not** aware of at my conscious level of awareness that is preventing me from
releasing my excess weight?   YES ___   NO ___

If YES, am I emotionally ready to know what that experience was?   YES ___   NO ___

If YES, can I deal with it on my own?   YES ___   NO ___

If the answer is NO to either of the above questions, do I need to consult a professional counselor?
YES ___   NO ___

*If you feel you are emotionally ready to know what the experience was and you are ready to deal with it on
your own, continue on. If at any point you feel the information is too traumatic or is more than you can
emotionally handle, stop answering the questions, turn your player back on and complete the session.*

What happened? _____
_____

How old was I? _____   Was anyone else involved?   YES ___   NO ___

If YES, who? _____

When and where did it happen? _____

Did it happen more than once?   YES ___   NO ___

Did I tell anyone about that experience?   YES ___   NO ___

If NO, why not? _____

If YES, who? _____

What was their reaction? _____

Why have I been suppressing that experience?   (Check all that apply.).

_____ It was traumatic

_____ It was embarrassing

_____ I feel guilty

_____ I feel responsible

_____ I should have known better

_____ It was not my fault, but I was told that it was

_____ It was not my fault, but I feel like it was

_____ Other _____

What do I need to do to release the effects of that experience and move on with my life? _____

_____

If I didn't have the excess weight would I feel vulnerable and exposed?   YES ___   NO ___

Besides my weight, what other areas of my life are being affected by that experience? _____

_____

Has that experience affected how I relate to the opposite sex?   YES ___   NO ___
If YES, how? _____

Has that experiences affected how I feel about myself?   YES ___   NO ___
If YES, how? _____

What do I need to do to release the effects of that experience and move on with my life? _____

_____

What are the best things that could happen if I stop suppressing and internalizing that experience? _____

_____

_____

Turn your CD player back on and relax as you listen to the suggestions that will help you release the effects of these experiences so you can move on with your life.

Wrap-Up

CONGRATULATIONS – YOU HAVE COMPLETED "TAKING ACTION" - ONE OF THE MOST IMPORTANT SECTIONS IN THIS PROGRAM. Weigh and measure yourself and chart your progress.

At this point in the program, you might feel your motivation slipping. If so, listen to the *"Let's Make An Agreement"* recording for several days in addition to the *"Set Yourself Free"* recording. Remember, you are not going to have to do this forever.

Just a reminder – reading your *"Weight Loss Agreement"* every day will also increase your motivation and commitment and will help erase any resistance you have to making positive changes in your life.

The focus of this section was to come to the understanding of how your emotions affect your physical and mental well-being. The written exercises and the *"Set Yourself Free"* recording were designed to help you identify and release your suppressed emotions.

You were also introduced to affirmations and how to use them to change your thinking and your life. They are a very powerful tool in creating your new, more positive reality. Utilize this new tool every chance you get. If you are creating your own affirmations, be sure to state them in the present tense (I am, I have) as an already accomplished fact.

"Mental Exercise 5" is one of the most important mental exercises in this program. It was designed to help you not only identify and resolve issues and experiences you may be aware of that could be affecting you weight, but also to discover the deeper underlying issues that could be affecting your ability to lose weight permanently. Repeating this exercise will be very beneficial, as you most likely initially encountered resistance to uncovering your deeper repressed issues.

If you are short of time and unable to physically exercise, listen to a recording and do the reading each day, try at least to listen to one of the recordings. Just be sure to not skip any of the reading or written exercises as everything included in this program is important and is designed to help you progress toward the achievement of your goal. Remind yourself you are making permanent life style changes that will improve your appearance and your health. It will become easier as your progress. You will soon find you are automatically making the choices that will insure your slim and healthy future.

Sometimes those things we fear in darkness
lose their power when brought
into the light of day

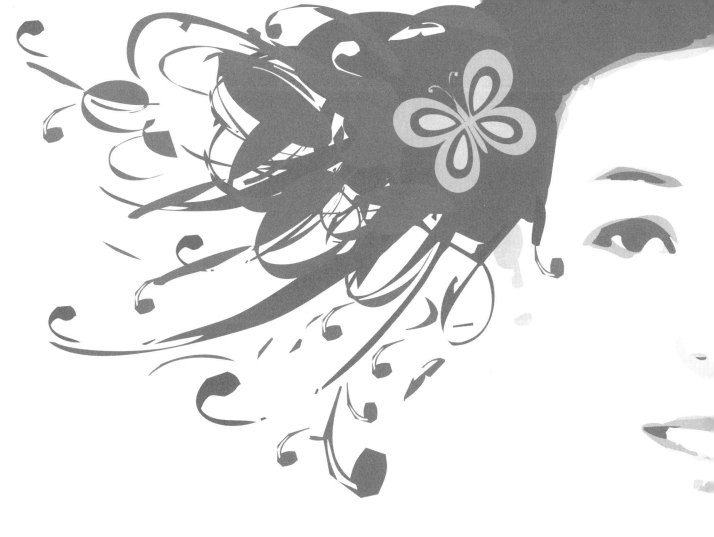

Releasing Past Programs

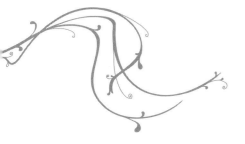

Releasing Past Programs

*By looking back we are
able to move forward!*

Were you required to eat every single thing on your plate before leaving the table, rewarded with food for your accomplishments or comforted with sweets when you hurt? If you still feel you have to clean your plate before leaving the table, celebrate your accomplishments with food, and sooth your hurts with sweets, you are responding to your childhood programming.

Do you feel compelled to eat when you're not really hungry? A need to eat for reasons other than nutritional needs are stimulated by your subconscious mind and may be the result of commercial programming, childhood messages, beliefs and cultural conditioning.

The written and mental exercises in this section will help you understand the connection you have with food and the emotional satisfaction you crave. Once you understand why you overeat and the deeper motivations that may be causing your attachment to food, you can break the connection between food and your emotions.

As a child you desired to be nurtured and loved. You desired to be a child, to play like a child and to slowly grow and mature into responsible adulthood. Perhaps a situation required you to grow up too fast, hold back your child-like responses, always "look good" and "be good," or to be "serious" and act like an adult. If so, your "Inner Child" withdrew so you could appear more responsible, serious, and achievement oriented. She was damaged and she needs to be healed.

Who is your "Inner Child?" What role does she play in your everyday decisions? What are the consequences of suppressing her?

You will connect with her and find out what she needs from you and how she can help you. "*Mental Exercise 6*" will help you discover the role she may be playing in your battle to gain control of your weight.

As you address and heal the deeper reasons for your behavior, you will heal and replace your old behavior with a new healthy lifestyle that will last for a lifetime!

Affirmations List

Read this list every day until you complete this section. Read each statement slowly and emphasize the bold, underlined words. Repeat each statement with conviction and the belief they are your reality.

- I **am** releasing the conditions of the past that have caused me to be overweight

- I have the **power** and **ability** to control my weight

- I **easily** attain and maintain my ideal weight

- I eat **smaller** portions at meals

- I **deserve** to be slender and healthy

- I have the **right** to be slim

- **Everything** I eat turns to health and vitality

- I **desire only** the amount of food required to keep me healthy and mentally alert

- I **choose** to leave food on my plate

- I **choose** to eat only at mealtime

- I **release** my emotions in a positive way

- I **choose** to be free of feeling deprived

- I **always** eat slowly

- I **know** what is good for me at all times

- I **love** myself **unconditionally**

- I **am** eating healthier and enjoying it more

- It's **OK** for me to leave food on my plate

- **Everything** I eat makes me slimmer and healthier **NOW**

- A slim and healthy body **is** my reality

Note: Read this list of affirmations every day for the next 10 days. Repeat each statement with conviction and the belief they are becoming your reality.

Your Inner Child

Carl Jung called her the "Divine Child" and Emmet Fox called her the "Wonder Child."

She is your "Inner Child" because of her child-like qualities. Sometimes she wants to play when you have to work. She pouts or throws a temper tantrum when she doesn't get her way. She wants to eat sweets when you have all but eliminated them from your list of acceptable foods. And she feels rejected if you don't pay enough attention to her and her needs.

You may prefer to give her another name. No matter what you call her, you were born with her and she will always be with you. She is your emotional self – she is where your feelings live. She is another voice from within that is guiding and directing you in many areas of your life.

When you were born she was fun loving, light hearted and happy. She had the seeds to be emotional and sensitive, creative, imaginative and artistic and to have fun and play for play's sake. She needed to feel loved and she needed to feel she was safe and secure.

The belief systems you developed as a child are also her beliefs and have been responsible for many of your experiences throughout your life.

If you grew up in a normal home where your needs were met, where you felt loved, nurtured and cared for, where you were encouraged to express yourself, where you had role models that showed you how to find pleasure in the "little" things in life, then it's more likely than not the seeds grew and you have grown into a confident, self assured woman who is not afraid to let her "Inner Child" come out and play.

However, you may have grown up in a dysfunctional family and your "Inner Child" is no longer the fun loving, free spirit she was when you were born. She was wounded, she was ignored, she was condemned and criticized, and she was confused. She withdrew and hid in order to survive in her world of stress.

If you were physically or sexually abused she withdrew even further and is still suffering. It is your "Inner Child" (not the adult you) who experiences the pain of being unworthy, the overwhelming feelings of guilt, the panic, terror, rage and hopelessness.

She is insecure, frightened and needy. She is afraid to take risks and needs encouragement every step of the way. She is the innocent child who has not been heard and is still waiting to hear that she is loved, that she is okay and she is "good enough."

Your childhood emotional wounds have been dictating your life and have kept you from loving yourself. They are underlying your anxiety, fear, confusion, emptiness and unhappiness. Until you connect with your "Inner Child" she will continue to feel isolated and alone. It's up to you to reclaim your childlike feelings, sensitivity, and wonderment.

It's never too late to have a happy childhood

Meeting Your Inner Child

It's not too late for the wise and loving woman you've become to meet and heal your "Inner Child." You can start building a loving relationship with her right now. You can offer her comfort and support and as you do you will find a new joy and energy in living.

The following process will help you meet and heal your "Child Within." It's a wonderful process that you can do over and over again. As you do this exercise, emotions you have been suppressing may begin to surface. If you feel like you need to cry, go ahead, the tears will cleanse and heal you.

Read this through to the end before you begin the process.

Choose a time and location where you can be undisturbed for about twenty to thirty minutes. Turn on some meditative music, find a comfortable position and begin by slowly relaxing each part of your body and mind. As you take nice slow deep breaths, filling your lungs slowly and completely before slowly exhaling, begin to imagine yourself in a beautiful, peaceful, safe and serene setting. As your body and mind relax, feel yourself being surrounded by peace and love.

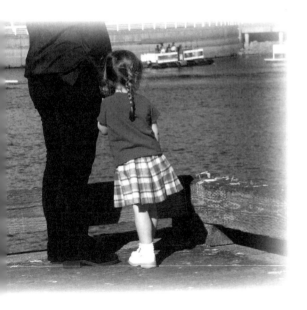

In your mind, picture a setting where you and your "Inner Child" can meet and get to know each other. Perhaps it's a private room where you will not be disturbed, where you can sit next to each other on a sofa or bed. You may choose a natural setting such as the beach or mountains where you may spread a blanket on the ground where you can sit and talk. You may choose to walk together, holding hands. Once you have created the setting, invite your "Inner Child" to join you.

Remember she has been hurt and ignored and she may be afraid of you or afraid to come out of her hiding place. She may appear immediately or it may take some time for her to feel comfortable enough to show herself to you. Coax her gently with love and understanding. Talk to her as you would a frightened child. Let her know you love her and want to get to know her. Let her know you are happy she is there and that you won't hurt her. Ask her to tell you what she wants and needs from you.

If she doesn't start talking to you, you can talk to her about anything that comes into your mind. Let her know that you are going to take care of her and you are not going to let anyone hurt her ever again.

When you feel you have completed the communications, embrace her with love and a warm, melting hug. Let her know you are leaving now, but you will always be there for her whenever she needs you. See her playfully leaving this peaceful scene you created.

When you are ready, gently come back to full awareness, bringing with you all the knowledge you gained from this exercise. Write in a journal as much as you can remember.

If you have difficulty picturing your "Inner Child," find some pictures of yourself between the ages of two and five. After you become familiar with how you looked, try again. You can also ask her to describe herself to you. How old she is? How tall is she? What color is her hair? What is she wearing?

What if she doesn't look like you looked? What you perceive is how she wants you to see her.

Whatever you do, DON'T give up! Keep trying. The process will become easier the more you do it.

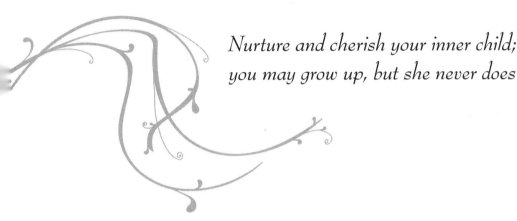

Nurture and cherish your inner child;
you may grow up, but she never does

Choose a time and location where you can be undisturbed for at least 20 minutes. If possible have your CD player within easy reach so you can pause it when instructed to do so during the exercise.

Listen to CD II – Track 3 and mentally ask yourself the following questions when instructed to do so. **Trust the first answer that comes into your mind** and write it in the space provided.

Mental Exercise 6

To heal the present you must go back and heal the past. Your "Inner Child" needs to be heard, to be liberated from under layers of conditioning, to know that she is safe and loved. Connecting with her will help you learn to experience from your inner self, the intimacy and the ability to communicate and express what is on your mind.

Drawing from your previous experience of getting in touch with your "Inner Child," complete the following:

Describe your "Inner Child" _____
_____
_____
_____
_____
_____

What does my "Inner Child" need from me? _____
_____
_____
_____

My "Inner Child" **feels**:

_____ Abused	_____ Happy	_____ Loved
_____ Angry	_____ Ignored	_____ Neglected
_____ Anxious	_____ Insecure	_____ Proud
_____ Confident	_____ Joyful	_____ Secure
_____ Frightened	_____ Lonely	_____ Unloved

My "Inner Child" protects herself from the pain when she is hurting with things like:

_____ Drugs	_____ Alcohol
_____ Food	_____ Cigarettes
_____ Work	_____ Relationships

My "Inner Child" **was**:

_____ Abandoned and she is fearful she will be abandoned again.
(She is starving for attention and reassurance and needs to feel safe and wanted)

_____ Neglected and doesn't feel she is lovable or worthwhile
(She is depressed and wants to hide and cry)

_____ Discounted and ignored
(She feels invisible and doesn't believe in herself)

_____ Taught she must always be doing something "worthwhile"
(She has forgotten how to be playful, creative, and spontaneous without guilt)

My "Inner Child" **is**:

_____ Spoiled and wants instant gratification
(She throws a temper tantrum when she doesn't get her own way)

_____ Anxious and in panic mode much of the time
(She has been overly criticized and needs lots of encouragement and positive affirmations)

_____ Disconnected, isolated and dissociated
(She has trouble trusting and has never been close to anyone)

What has my "Inner Child" done to get my attention? *Example: Being bad or naughty, overeating.*

1. _____
2. _____
3. _____
4. _____

What is my "Inner Child" trying to get me to hear? *Example: I'm scared. I need you.*

1. _____
2. _____
3. _____
4. _____

What messages did my "Inner Child" need to hear that were never said? *Example: I love you. I care about you.*

1. _____
2. _____
3. _____
4. _____

My "Inner Child" is hungry for:

1. _____
2. _____
3. _____
4. _____

I can give my "Inner Child" the following nurturing messages:

1. _____
2. _____
3. _____
4. _____

Turn your CD player back on and relax as you listen to the suggestions that will assist you in reaching your weight goal.

Exposing Deeper Needs and Excuses for Overeating

We all have the desire and drive for food and eating. It's a natural instinct we were born with and we could not survive without it. When this desire and drive goes beyond the normal physical need our body has for nutrition, it may be a manifestation of conditioning.

To slim people, food is nothing more than food,
no matter how delicious, enjoyable,
elegantly served, or charming the
company at the dinner table

You may think you want to be slim, yet you find yourself compelled to indulge in unhealthy foods or simply overeat. This behavior is fulfilling deeper needs. Those deeper needs may represent attempts to compensate for a lack of love, feeling inadequate or incomplete, or for a deficiency in any area of your life. This may have been conditioned into you through cultural, commercial, or family programming. Advertisers are especially adept at capitalizing on your feelings of lack and replacing them with the false idea that a product can fill the empty space within you.

Food may be a symbol of warmth, comfort, security, reward, stimulation, sedation, and sex. Overeating may be an expression of your anger or an attempt to suppress it. It may be a way for you to sustain physical and emotional distance or a form of self-punishment.

The purpose of the following exercises is to bring to your conscious awareness the subconscious motivations that may be causing you to follow unhealthy eating patterns. Once you understand the subconscious needs you are satisfying, you can consciously take control and make the proper choices and decisions regarding your eating patterns.

Take your time with this exercise. Read each statement slowly and really think about whether it applies to you. This is your opportunity to get in touch with more of the reasons you have not been able to release your excess weight. Be open to this process and be aware of even the slightest thought, feeling or emotion that might connect you to the statement.

Place an "A" for <u>ALWAYS</u>, "S" for <u>SOMETIMES</u> or "N" <u>NEVER</u> next to each statement. Be honest with yourself, for only by being honest can you release yourself and move forward.

Food as a Reward

As a child your parents may have rewarded you with candy or treats for good grades, good behavior, or a job well done. As an adult you may be continuing to reward yourself for completing a task on time, a good days work, a promotion, getting a new customer, or just getting through a difficult day.

_____ I reward myself with food for my accomplishments.

Food as a Substitute for Love or Affection

You may be using food to cure your hurts or fulfill your longing for love. You may be attempting to fill the emptiness or block out the emotional pain of an unhappy relationship by overindulging in food.

_____ I lack love or a close relationship in my life. I use food to fill the void.

_____ I am falling out of love, or someone is falling out of love with me. That relationship is causing me to feel upset, confused, anxious, angry and hurt. I use food to sooth the hurt and block my pain.

_____ I was the child of a working mother who never seemed to have enough time to give me the attention I needed. I accepted food as a replacement for the love and affection that was missing in my life.

_____ Whenever I feel unloved or don't receive enough attention or affection, I eat.

Overeating = Overweight = Look at Me

We all need attention from the people we love and we will often go to great lengths to get it. If this need is great enough we will go to any extent, even to negative attention to meet our needs.

_____ I need more recognition and affection from the people in my life. If I am "bigger" they will have to notice me.

Overeating = Overweight = Please Don't Notice Me

Are you shy? Do you lack confidence in your ability to interact in social situations? Would you rather people didn't notice you?

_____ I want to be anonymous. If I am "bigger" people might not pay attention to me.

Personal Power

Do you equate weight with power and strength? Does being slim or looking feminine represent weakness? Deep down you may be confusing physical weight with "weight of influence."

_____ I will not be as powerful and influential if I am slim.

Overeating As a Means of Escaping a Disagreeable Life Situation

A sensation similar to drinking alcohol is created when you overeat. The excess food sits in your stomach and ferments and while your body is attempting to process this excess food you can experience sensations of drowsiness, numbness, and general loss of energy, which helps to insulate you from your feelings.

_____ I have a nagging spouse, parent or employer. I eat more than my body can assimilate in an attempt to escape from the situation.

_____ I eat to escape or forget about my worries and anxieties.

Food Is Comforting

As an infant you may have been given the breast or formula when you cried, regardless of what was causing your discomfort. As a child your mother may have given you cookies or candy when you hurt yourself or were upset, telling you that it would make you feel better. You began to make an association between food and comfort that you may have carried with you into adulthood. You may have become so accustomed to using food to erase tension, anxiety, pain, frustration and other emotional symptoms you may now be attempting to solve all of your problems by eating.

_____ I automatically reach for food if I have had a quarrel with a loved one, been reprimanded by my boss, lost my job, or need to be comforted.

I'm an Adult, I'll Eat What I Want

When you were a child your parents exerted a great deal of control over what you ate. If you were forced to eat foods you didn't want, you may have gotten angry and rebelled, adopting the view "When I grow up, I'll eat whatever I want, whenever I want."

_____ I am proving no one else can control what I eat by rejecting the "have to eats" of my childhood and eating all of the "No No's."

I'll Do It My Way

We all need to have some independence in our life and we often resort to extreme measures to achieve it.

_____ I have an extremely dominating person in my life always telling me what to do. I feel they may control my life but I won't let them control my body.

I'm Getting Even

Parents and other people we love often place great importance on personal appearance. Do you have a reason for revenge? Neglecting your body can be a great way of getting even.

_____ I am trying to "get even" with _____ by being overweight.

Relationship Barriers

Meeting new people and participating in social functions can be frightening. Extending yourself in friendship sets you up for rejection. Becoming involved in a close relationship can be painful. Are those extra pounds your way of keeping people from getting too close to you?

_____ I am afraid of being rejected or hurt.

Missing Mother

Did you grow up without a mother, or did your mother ignore you and your needs. Are you filling that need by mothering yourself?

_____ I mother myself with food.

The Motherly Image

What image do you normally conjure up when you think of Mom? Is it the ultra-slim, sexy model on the cover of Cosmopolitan magazine? Probably not! Subconsciously, you think of a soft, warm, ample lap to sit on and full, nurturing breasts. In other words a plump unassuming woman who neglects her own needs while being interested only in the welfare of her children.

_____ I am a mother and physically reflecting the motherly image.
_____ I play the role of "mother" for my spouse.

Anger Suppression

Were you taught as a child that anger was an inappropriate emotion and should not be expressed? Anger is a healthy response in certain situations and suppressing it means that it stays locked up inside and can lead to overeating as an attempt to cover it up.

_____ I internalize my anger rather than expressing or exposing it.

_____ I attempt to work out my anger by subconsciously choosing to eat hard, tough foods that I can bite or tear apart.

_____ I am afraid to show my anger and I choose soft, mushy foods that cannot be linked to hard, emotional, angry chewing.

He Who Hesitates

Did you come from a large family where you frequently had to take your food and eat it fast, because if you didn't someone else would. This environment frequently establishes a subconscious need to "sneak" food and eat fast.

_____ I am the product of a large family and I am still eating as if someone will get the food before I do.

Weight As a Barrier to Sexual Fulfillment

Many facets of sexuality are reflected through overeating. Gaining weight to be less attractive to the opposite sex is a common occurrence for both single and married individuals. It is a subconscious solution to avoiding sexual encounters. It may reflect a fear or dislike for the sexual experience as the result of incest or rape, or may be an attempt to insure marital fidelity by limiting the opportunities to be unfaithful.

_____ I am afraid of sexual encounters.

_____ I am afraid the opposite sex will be more attracted to me if I lose weight.

_____ I am afraid I may lose control and give in to all kinds of sexual opportunities if I lose weight.

Yearning For Fulfillment

Most parents receive satisfaction and gratification from raising and taking care of their children. Meeting their needs is rewarding and fulfilling. What do you do to receive the same pleasure and satisfaction when they no longer depend upon you to meet their needs? Have you recently retired or quit a job that gave you a great deal of satisfaction? Are you looking for the same kind of compensation from eating? Eating to fill the void in your life is only a temporary measure and does not satisfy the underlying emotional desire to be needed.

_____ I have a void in my life I try to satisfy with food.

_____ I look for compensation when I eat.

_____ I have been meeting other people's needs for so long I have forgotten how to fulfill my own.

Food and Relaxation

Do you drive yourself hard and stop only when you have to eat? Do you feel guilty when you are not working or if you take time out to relax? You may be associating food and relaxation.

_____ Eating is my excuse to kick back and relax for a few minutes.

Role Model

Did you have a favorite grandparent, aunt, uncle or cousin that you vowed to be "just like" when you grew up? Were they overweight? If you wanted to be just like them and they weighed 250 pounds, you may have modeled your body after them. The reverse of this situation may also be true. If you had a poor relationship with someone close to you, you may have resolved to be nothing like them? Were they slim? You may have rejected everything about them, including their slim body.

_____ I had an overweight "idol" when I was young and I am trying to be just like them.

_____ I had a poor relationship with my mother or father and I reject everything about them, including their slender body.

The "Poor Starving Children" Syndrome

If you cannot bear to see food wasted and you must eat every last scrap on your plate, whether or not you are hungry, it's probably the result of a childhood program that instructed you to "Think of the poor starving children in _____." As an adult this statement echoes in your mind when you approach the end of a meal, and you feel guilty if you don't finish the last mouthful.

_____ I cannot leave food on my plate and feel good about it.

Food to Relieve Boredom

Do you have more time on your hands than you know what to do with? Have you developed rituals of planning, shopping, preparing, eating and cleaning up to fill your idle time?

_____ I am bored and I plan and prepare elaborate decadent meals to fill my time.

_____ I eat because it gives me something to do.

Food Keeps You Healthy

"You look so thin dear, are you sick?" Many people connect weight loss with illness and death, and extra pounds with survival. Many illnesses result in weight loss and have nothing to do with your diet or how much you weigh.

As an infant or young child were you ill, very thin, or did you almost die? Did someone close to you lose a lot of weight before they died?

_____ I associate health with extra pounds.

_____ I have a fear of becoming thin and dying.

Prosperity

In many cultures the fat look has represented abundance, riches and wealth. Loading the table with an abundance of rich food can be a carryover from this type of prosperity thinking, and may be the reflection of a meager childhood.

_____ I bring home lots of goodies and serve large, rich meals.

_____ I think of my weight as a reflection of my cultural beliefs

Just Because

It's there, it's time, it looks good, or it smells good. You may eat at certain times or under certain circumstances that have nothing to do with your stomach telling you it's hungry. Do you frequently join the office "lunch bunch" even though you may not be hungry, just so you won't be left out? When you see other people eating do you get hungry and eat too.

_____ I am caught up in the "lunch time ritual."

_____ I eat with others just to be sociable.

_____ I eat when I'm not hungry

_____ The sight, thought, or smell of food makes my mouth water.

Deeper Needs Exposed

For each of the "A" statements, choose an alternative activity to eating that could possibly meet your subconscious needs and write them below.

1. _____
2. _____
3. _____
4. _____
5. _____
6. _____
7. _____
8. _____
9. _____
10. _____

For each of the "S" statements, choose an alternative activity to eating that could possibly meet your subconscious needs and write them below.

1. _____
2. _____
3. _____
4. _____
5. _____
6. _____
7. _____
8. _____
9. _____
10. _____

Become aware of those times when you are eating to satisfy subconscious rather than physical needs and chooses an alternative activity instead of eating.

Conditioned Responses

Y ou have certain eating patterns and routines that have been instilled over a period of time. You may have already discovered some of them may go as far back as your childhood. These act as conditioned stimulus and result in your eating when you are not physically hungry. As a result of this conditioning, going to certain places, doing certain things or being with certain people automatically stimulates your urge to eat.

The first step in changing your reactive eating patterns is to identify those times and activities that stimulate you to eat. Watching television, reading a book, preparing food, watching other people eat, being alone and doing housework are a few of the activities that can act as triggers for arousing an eating response.

To free yourself from these unnecessary urges, you must identify your conditioned responses and then work on changing your reactive patterns. You can do this by making eating an experience that is not associated with any other event.

It may be easier for you to be overweight
than to make the changes that
will improve your life

Exposing Conditioned Responses

Below, list those situations and activities that cause you to eat when you are not physically hungry. Next to the activity or situation, write an alternative activity to eating that will help you overcome your unhealthy conditioning.

Activity or Situation	**Alternative to Eating**
Example: Eating something sweet after a meal.	Example: I'll clean up the kitchen and brush my teeth

Experiencing certain emotions, situations and feelings can also trigger an eating response. Place a check mark next to any of the following you react to by eating.

_____ Happiness	_____ Sadness	_____ Rejection
_____ Fear	_____ Depression	_____ Failure
_____ Success	_____ Jealousy	_____ Loneliness
_____ Criticism	_____ Insecurity	_____ Feeling Inferior
_____ Sexual Pleasure	_____ Fatigue	_____ Anger
_____ Making Decisions	_____ Boredom	_____ Frustration
_____ Sexual Problems	_____ Stress	_____ Dreary Weather

Choose a time and location where you can be undisturbed for at least 20 minutes. If possible have your CD player within easy reach so you can pause it when instructed to do so during the exercise.

Listen to CD II – Track 3 and mentally ask yourself the following questions when instructed to do so. **Trust the first answer that comes into your mind** and write it in the space provided.

Mental Exercise 7

In the memory banks of your subconscious mind are all of the childhood messages you received about food. These messages may prompt you to eat when you are not physically hungry. The purpose of this exercise is to make you aware of those childhood messages that are still controlling the way you react to food. Once again, listen for your inner voice and don't rush the answers.

Looking back over my life, who has been the most important influence in how I relate to food?

_____

As a child, what messages did I receive from my parents and other adults about eating? _____

_____

At what age did I accept those messages? _____

Which ones are still affecting how I relate to food today? _____

_____

Where do they fit into my life now? _____

_____

Why am I still accepting those messages? _____

_____

Turn your CD player back on and relax as you listen to the suggestions that will assist you in reaching your weight goal.

Excuses For Being Overweight

Make a list of the excuses you give yourself and others for not losing weight.
*Example: **"I'm too tired to exercise."***

_____

_____

_____

_____

_____

_____

_____

_____

_____

_____

Change each excuse into a positive affirmation and write them below.
*Example: **"I have an abundance of energy for exercising."***

_____

_____

_____

_____

_____

_____

_____

_____

_____

_____

Become aware of the excuses you use for not losing weight and each time you catch yourself making one of these excuses, change the negative into a positive statement and reinforce it by either writing it down several times or repeating it in your mind four or five times.

Payoffs for Being Overweight

Think about what you really get out of being overweight. Make a list of the payoffs you receive for being overweight. *Example:* *"I get to eat whatever I want, whenever I want."*

_____

_____

_____

_____

_____

_____

_____

_____

_____

_____

Change each payoff into a positive affirmation and write them below.
Example: I eat only at mealtimes and only the amount of food necessary to sustain me nutritionally.

_____

_____

_____

_____

_____

_____

_____

_____

_____

_____

Wrap-Up

CONGRATULATIONS – YOU HAVE JUST COMPLETED "RELEASING PAST PROGRAMS."
Weigh yourself and chart your progress. Do something good for yourself – you deserve it!

Uncovering your subconscious motivations can be a difficult and very emotional experience. Continuing to uncover and resolve these issues will be extremely valuable, as you will be releasing yourself from the hold they have had on you. This is a positive step toward taking back control of your responses to food.

If you find yourself making excuses for not working with this program on a daily basis, re-evaluate your desire, determination and commitment to achieving your goal. If you don't have enough time to exercise, do a reading topic and listen to a recorded program each day, work at a pace you can fit into your time schedule. Just be sure you do something every day and complete everything in this section before moving on to "*Self-Reflections & Self Love*." Just do what you can each day. The most important thing is to complete every step of this program, not how long it takes to do it.

Looking at your past
shows you the path to changing your future

The focus of this section was looking back at when and how you were programmed regarding food and the role it plays in your life. You also had the opportunity to meet and get to know your inner child. If you had trouble visualizing or connecting with her, keep trying. Be patient and let her know you love her and will protect her. She will come.

You also looked at your conditioned responses and how they trigger you to eat when you are not physically hungry. Identifying those times and activities is the first step to changing your reactive eating patterns.

Continue to monitor the excuses you use for not losing weight and each time you catch yourself making an excuse, change it into a positive statement. Reinforce your positive statement by writing it several times or repeating it in your mind four or five times.

"*Mental Exercise 7*" prompted you to recall the childhood messages you received about food. If they are messages that are contributing to your being overweight, look at them from your adult perspective and think about how you can release yourself from the hold they have had on you. AWARENESS is an important step to taking back control of your weight.

CONGRATULATE YOURSELF for the efforts you are making to change your life!

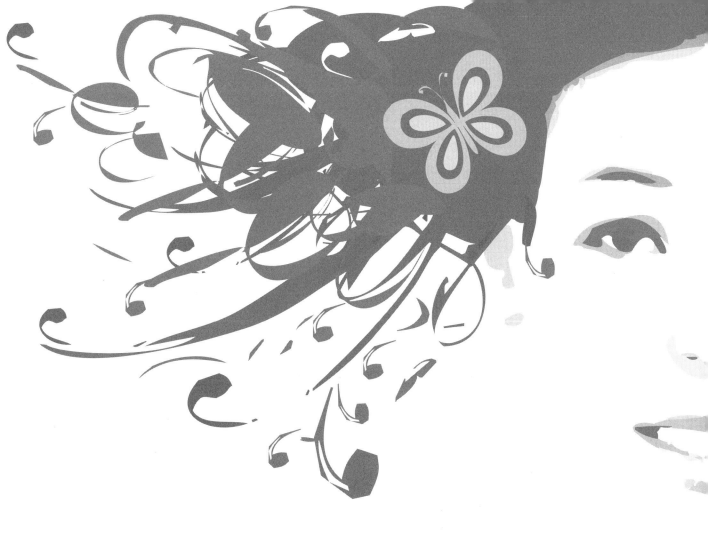

Self-Reflections & Self-Love

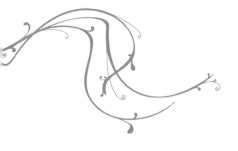

Self-Reflections & Self-Love

Find your love within and you will never be without!

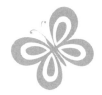

A few years ago Tina Turner recorded a popular song entitled "What's Love Got to Do With It." To take her title one step further, your theme song for this section will be entitled "What's Self-Love Got to Do With It?" And the answer is . . . . . EVERYTHING.

In current writings Self-Love and Self-Esteem seem to be interchangeable, but no matter which terminology feels comfortable to you, the experts agree that much of it is developed in the first three years of life and is based on the development of trust and unconditional parental love. Without it we move through life feeling unworthy or that we will never be good enough, lacking confidence, seeking approval of others, comparing ourselves to others, desperate to be in relationships. Without Self-Love we stay in abusive relationships, abuse addictive substances and overeat to escape our feelings.

Having Self-Love means that your well-being matters to you unconditionally and the more you have the better you treat yourself. Do you really love yourself, your family, your parents? Or is it that you want to love, but don't know how? No matter where you feel you are on a scale of 1 to 10, let's just say it can be improved.

Loving yourself begins with the acceptance of who you are at this very moment and gives you a foundation to build upon. As you progress through the exercises in this section, you will come to an understanding of how your concept of love developed and the "*Adventure in Self-Love*" recording will help you release your negative thoughts, criticisms and judgments about yourself. Listening to this recording on a daily basis as you progress through this section will help you replace the negatives with the positive feelings of self-acceptance, peace and your own self-love.

Before looking at your love and how you express it, you will do several more written exercises dealing with your negative suppressed emotions. You'll determine if you are still carrying heavy thoughts and burdens that could be contributing to your overweight.

After you put the negatives behind, you will be more receptive to focusing on love and acceptance and your own uniqueness.

Self Talk Revisited

In the "**Self Talk**" exercise (page 83) in the "**Self-Evaluation**" section, you made a list of the negative things you tell yourself about your appearance and you re-wrote each statement in positive terms that support the way you want to look after you reach your goal.

Are you still giving yourself negative suggestions about your appearance? If YES, write them below.

1. _____
2. _____
3. _____
4. _____
5. _____
6. _____
7. _____
8. _____
9. _____
10. _____

Change these negatives into positive statements and write them below.

1. _____
2. _____
3. _____
4. _____
5. _____
6. _____
7. _____
8. _____
9. _____
10. _____

Make a new list incorporating your new positive statements with your previous list of "**Positive Statements**." Make several copies of this new list. Replace the copy on your refrigerator with this new list, place a second copy where you will see it sometime during the day and place a third copy where you will remember to read it just before you go to bed.

Hate = Weight

Positive emotions, like the emotion of love, are light, free and flowing. Have you noticed, when you are in a positive frame of mind, you feel light, free, alive and enthusiastic about your life. You feel good about yourself and you look forward to your future.

Negative emotions, on the other hand, are "heavy" emotions and they can weigh you down and hold your back from becoming all you are capable of being. They also change the way you feel physically and emotionally. When you see things from a negative perspective, or harbor negative emotions, you experience feelings of tiredness, heaviness, or depression. You have no hope, no drive, no ambition. Your future looks dismal. These same negative emotions, when suppressed, can also transform into excess weight on your body.

Hate is one of these "heavy" negative emotions that is restrictive and can block the natural free flow of energy through your body, disturbing the harmony and balance of all of your bodily functions.

Do you despise or have a strong aversion or dislike for anyone? A portion of your excess weight could be the extreme dislike and hostility you are suppressing.

Make a list of those **people and situations you feel extreme dislike or hostility towards.** Include anyone who has caused you to suffer with unkind words, has physically or mentally abused you, or anyone you feel would like to get even with you.

Person or Situation	Reason

Make a list of the **people you have hurt or wronged**. Include anyone you have caused to suffer by your unkind words or anyone you would like to get even with.

Person   Reason

_____   _____

_____   _____

_____   _____

_____   _____

_____   _____

_____   _____

_____   _____

Your overweight could be a reflection of your own self-hate. What do you hate yourself for?

Listen to CD I – Track 3 and set yourself free.

Heavy Thoughts and Weight

Are you carrying "HEAVY" thoughts around with you, thoughts that may have manifested in physical weight? These could include financial burdens, responsibilities for parents, social obligations, self-imposed burdens (i.e. having to do everything perfectly), or feeling responsible or guilty for something that happened in the past.

Write down all of the burdens you are carrying around with you. List those things you are ashamed of or feel guilty about.

_____

_____

_____

_____

_____

_____

How could you make those burdens lighter?

_____

_____

_____

Could you release yourself completely from some of those burdens?   YES ___ NO ___

If YES, how would you feel and how would your life change if you released them? _____

_____

Would releasing those burdens make you feel lighter?   YES ___ NO ___

Love and Acceptance

Your image of yourself is based on how you feel about yourself from within. The person you see in the mirror is only a part of who you are. If you are like most overweight women, you look in the mirror and see all of the things you want to change and none of the things you feel are right about you.

Are you avoiding seeing all the beautiful things about yourself that others see? Do you look at yourself as if you were under a microscope, seeing every flaw, every imperfection? Does a small blemish look the size of a potato. Are your beautiful eyes never seen because you are focusing on the imperfectness you feel about yourself?

What do you see when you look at other women – surely not what they see every day when they are scrutinizing themselves. If you know them, you look past their imperfections to the core of who they are and you see their inner beauty.

HELLO! WAKE UP! You are beautiful too and you need to start seeing yourself as others who know and love you see you. They see the love you give to others. They see your devotion, your caring and your competence. They see your style, your charm, your special smile and the twinkle in your eyes. They feel the warmth of your hug, the love that radiates through the simple touch of your hand on theirs, and the feelings behind the thoughtful card you sent.

Who you are inside is more important than the wrinkles (smile lines) around your eyes, your hair that won't go the way you want it to in the morning, or the numbers you see when you step on the scale.

You have been your own worst enemy – It's
time to be your own best friend!

Loving and accepting yourself and your body is one of the most important gifts you can give to yourself and to those who love you. The more you love and accept yourself the more love you will be able to give to others and the more quickly you will become the physical person you desire to see in the mirror.

Take some time to think about each question below before writing your answers.

Write your definition of love.

_____

_____

Write your definition of self-love.

_____

_____

Write your definition of acceptance.

_____

_____

Now, go to the dictionary and look up the definitions for **love**, **self** and **acceptance.** Write a new definition for **self-love** incorporating all of the definitions.

_____

_____

_____

I'll give you a little help – it might go something like this – "A profoundly tender, passionate affection toward your nature and character, just as you are right now, with all of your perceived faults and shortcomings."

Can you begin to love and accept yourself within the context of your new definition of self-love?
YES ___ NO ___

If NO, why not? _____

_____

What would have to change before you could say YES and mean it? _____

_____

Do you feel other people love and accept you? YES ___ NO ___

Do you think other people would love and accept you more if you were at your ideal weight?
YES ___ NO ___

If yes, why do you think you would be more accepted and more lovable? _____

_____

To Love and Be Loved

Do you feel loved? The lack of love is something we all feel from time to time, but when it becomes persistent it is often described as a "feeling of emptiness" and we may try to fill the void with food.

Make a list of the people who love and care about you.

_____   _____

_____   _____

_____   _____

_____   _____

List some of the things these people do for you to show you they love and care about you.

_____

_____

_____

Make a list of the people **you** really love and care about.

_____   _____

_____   _____

_____   _____

_____   _____

Llist some of the things you do for others to show them you love and care about them.

_____

_____

_____

List some of the things you do for yourself because you love yourself.

_____

_____

_____

I Am Special

A. Make a list of the things you would like someone to do for you that would make you feel cared about and special. ***Example: Send me flowers.***

_____

_____

_____

_____

_____

B. Make a list of personal things you could do for yourself that would make you feel good and would be an expression of self-love. ***Example: Get a massage!***

_____

_____

_____

_____

_____

C. Make a list of the statements you would like someone in your family to say to you that would make you feel "special" and loved. ***Example: "I really appreciate what you do for me."***

_____

_____

_____

_____

_____

D. If you work, make a list of statements or comments you would like your employer, supervisor or co-workers to say to you that would make you feel your work is noticed and appreciated.
Example: "You really did a good job on that project."

_____

_____

_____

_____

_____

E. Make a list of things you would like to do in your primary relationship that would make your relationship special. ***Example: Plan a special "date" for no reason.***

_____

_____

_____

_____

_____

F. Make a list of things you would like to do for your body that would be an expression of self-love. ***Example: Exercise.***

_____

_____

_____

_____

_____

Question: Did you list five things in each section? If not, go back and finish each section. If you can't think of five things, think about what you would do for your best friend. Think of the things you say to your best friend to make them feel good. Complete your list with these things.

Choose your favorite one from each of the above sections and write it below.

A. _____

B. _____

C. _____

D. _____

E. _____

F. _____

Note: *For item C, write yourself a "special" note as if it came from someone in your family. For item D, write yourself a note of appreciation related to your work. Mail your "special" notes to yourself at your home address.*

DO each one of the remaining items for yourself as soon as possible. - YOU DESERVE IT.

Success List

Make a list of your past and present achievements. Include the small as well as the significant accomplishments. These could include any awards you have received, fears you have overcome and goals you have accomplished.

My Past Achievements

_____

_____

_____

My Present Achievements

_____

_____

_____

Defining your goals for the future is an important first step in bringing those goals to reality. Make a list of those things that you desire to be your future accomplishments. Achieving your weight goal should be at the top of your list.

My Future Achievements

_____

_____

_____

Choose a time and location where you can be undisturbed for at least 20 minutes. If possible have your CD player within easy reach so you can pause it when instructed to do so during the exercise.

Listen to CD II – Track 3 and mentally ask yourself the following questions when instructed to do so. **Trust the first answer that comes into your mind** and write it in the space provided.

Mental Exercise 8

Your concept of love began to develop the day you were born and has continued to change and develop through your life in response to your ever changing personal relationships. The following questions will help you better understand where you learned about love and how it relates to how you feel about yourself and your self-esteem.

Whose ideas of love did I accept? _____

How old was I? _____

What did they teach me about love and self-acceptance? _____
_____

From my adult perspective, were they good ideas and in my best interest?   YES ___   NO ___

How have I incorporated those ideas of love into the way I feel about myself? _____
_____

How have I incorporated those ideas of love into my personal relationships? _____
_____

Have my ideas of love changed?   YES ___   NO ___

If YES, how have they changed? _____
_____

Why have they changed? _____

_____

How would my life be different if I loved and accepted myself more? _____

_____

What are my greatest strengths? _____

What are my weaknesses? _____

How can I overcome those weaknesses? _____

_____

Why is self-love important? _____

_____

Turn your CD player back on and relax as you listen to the suggestions that will assist you in reaching your weight goal.

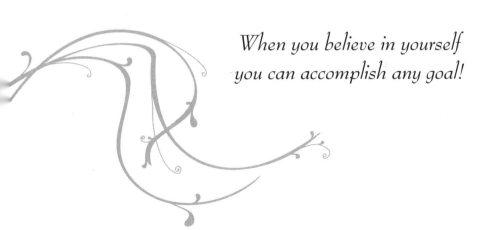

*When you believe in yourself
you can accomplish any goal!*

Self Drawing - Part 1

Have you been going through life only looking in a mirror to put on your makeup or comb your hair, avoiding looking at the rest of your body? This indicates you are ashamed or embarrassed about your overweight.

Please don't skip this exercise because you are uncomfortable with how you think you look. This exercise is important because it will indicate how you perceive yourself. You will discover in a later exercise whether your perception is accurate.

In the box at the right, draw a picture that represents how you think you look at your present weight. Draw your size, shape and proportions as accurately as you can. It doesn't make any difference whether it is a front or back view. Don't use the excuse that you're not an artist or you don't know how to draw. It doesn't have to be perfect. What is important about this exercise is that you draw a representation of the way you think you look.

Wrap-Up

YOU HAVE JUST COMPLETED THE "SELF-REFLECTIONS & SELF-LOVE" SECTION OF THIS PROGRAM. CONGRATULATE YOURSELF FOR YOUR COMMITMENT. Every exercise you complete is moving you closer to the slim person you desire to be. Weigh and measure yourself and chart your progress.

The first exercise in this section has you checking in to see if you are still giving yourself negative suggestions about yourself and your appearance. When you are working on making positive changes in your life, it's very easy to slip back into those old habit patterns that have been established over a long period of time. Continue to monitor your self talk and immediately change any negative to a positive. As you continue to do this you will notice that you will have to do it less and less as your new positive way of thinking replaces your old habit pattern.

You were also introduced to the "weight" of negative emotions and how they can affect your physical weight. The more you release your negative thoughts, feelings, and emotions the more positive your life will become and the more easily you will reach and maintain your ideal weight.

Self-Love – how important is it? Very important! If we lived in a perfect world we would have grown up in a family that understood how important it is to feel loved and accepted and they would have done everything they could to make sure that we grew up full of self-love and self-esteem. Unfortunately, we don't live in a perfect world and our childhood years may have left us feeling empty inside and not knowing why or how to fill the emptiness. For you, food may be your attempt to fill the emptiness. The *"Adventure in Self-Love"* recording will help you begin to replace any feeling of emptiness with self-acceptance and love, your own self-love.

Whether you think so or not, **you are special** and you need to start treating yourself with the love and respect you deserve. When you believe you are special and deserving, other people will too, and your life will be forever changed.

Love is the light that
illuminates your path through life

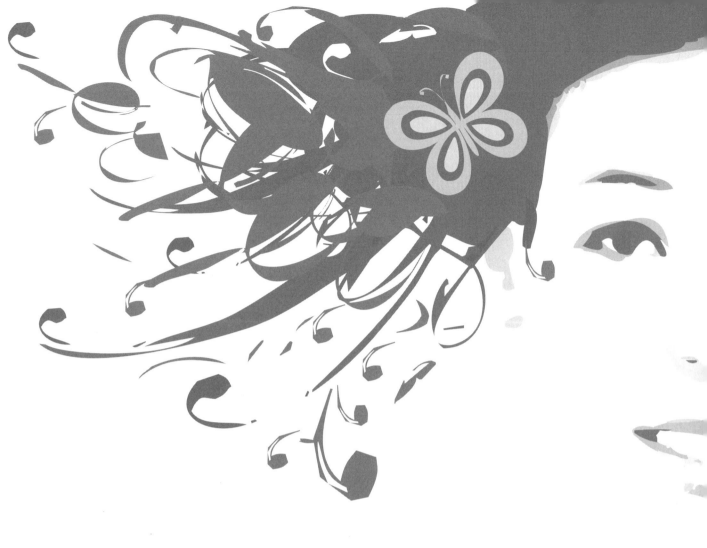

Looking Forward, The New You

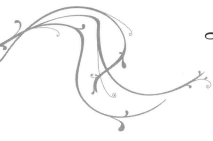

Looking Forward, The New You

There is a beautiful butterfly inside of you waiting to emerge!

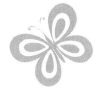

Welcome to the "New You." This section is all about the person you are and the person you are in the process of becoming.

Most people do not come with a simple switch that they can flip to change their behavior. All of our behaviors have an origin, no matter how complex they may seem. When we dig deep and uncover the reasons for our behaviors, we are able to realize change within ourselves.

How well do you know yourself? Have you ever really stopped to think about who you really are? What wonderful qualities do you possess that makes you special, unique and different from everyone else on this planet? What areas of your personality could you change that would make you a better person?

Genuine self-reflection affects so many aspects of your life – the presence of gratitude, your relationships with your loved ones, the degree of judgment you place on other's faults, your mental health and lifestyle choices.

The first exercise in this section, "*Soul Searching*," will give you the opportunity to look at all of your behaviors realistically and from a detached perspective. The first step is a willingness to honestly face your mistakes, deficiencies, failures, transgressions and actions which have caused difficulty to others. When you are able to accept those less acceptable behaviors, you can begin to move forward and let go of the pain. When the burden of the past is lifted, you can replace your former behaviors with loving actions. When this happens, you will transform your life and the lives of those close to you.

You will continue to focus on self-love through the written exercises of "*The Unique Me*" and "*Who Am I*."

Did you do the "*Self Drawing Part 1*" exercise in the last section? If NO, go back and complete it because you need it to complete "*Self Drawing – Part 2.*"

"*Mental Exercise 9*" will project you to the future when your ideal body is your reality and you will be able assess your progress up to this point.

Listen to "*The New You*" recording, alternating with the "*Adventure In Self-Love*" recording while completing this section.

With every step on your journey, you are becoming "The New You."

Soul Searching

As human beings we have a desire to know ourselves and to find meaning in our lives. We may be the only creatures on earth who can observe our own thoughts and feelings and recall the actions and events of the past as if observing ourselves in a mirror. Unfortunately, all too often, we are victims of ego-delusion. Our minds are continually dominated by an endless train of egocentric thoughts of greed, attachment, anger, pride, envy and passion, rather than the uplifting thoughts of love, tolerance, compassion, peace and forgiveness that lead to happier and more meaningful lives.

A sincere examination of yourself is not an easy task. It requires you to look at all of your behaviors realistically and from a totally detached perspective. It involves a willingness to honestly face your mistakes, deficiencies, failures, transgressions and actions which have caused difficulty to others, rather than just your positive traits, characteristics and behaviors.

Once again, this exercise will only be of value if you are truthful with yourself.

Check each of the following that represent an aspect of who you are or the way you respond.

___ I don't mind being wrong.	___ I am always right.
___ I look for ways to give to others.	___ I have thoughts of greed.
___ I am happy when other people win.	___ I get angry when I lose.
___ I appreciate what I have.	___ I am envious of others.
___ I forgive those who I feel have hurt me.	___ I look for ways to get even when hurt.
___ I am generous towards others.	___ I am selfish.
___ I am confident about myself and my abilities.	___ I feel I am not as good as other people.
___ I accept it when I am wrong.	___ I am always right.
___ I accept responsibility when it's my fault.	___ It's always the other persons fault.
___ I look for valid criticisms so I can improve.	___ I'm perfect and don't need to improve.
___ I am a good loser.	___ If someone else wins I vow to get even.
___ I accept I'm not perfect.	___ I'm perfect and I don't need to change.
___ I trust everyone till I have reason not to.	___ I mistrust everyone.
___ I can change my view if the argument is good.	___ My view is the only truth.
___ I am no better or worse than anyone else.	___ I feel I am better than everyone else.
___ I am proud of myself.	___ I am prideful.
___ I am realistic about my faults & shortcomings.	___ I am overly critical of myself.
___ I feel worthy of having good things in my life.	___ I feel unworthy of experiencing good.
___ I love who I am.	___ I hate who I am.
___ I accept how I look and know I am changing.	___ I am disgusted with how I look.
___ I love myself unconditionally.	___ I can't love myself unconditionally.
___ I respect myself.	___ I have no respect for other people.
___ I respect other people.	___ I have no respect for myself.

1. What of yourself (your time, talent and energies) have you given to others? _____

_____

2. What have you received from others? _____

_____

3. What trouble have you caused others? List who, what and why you chose to do so.

_____

_____

4. What troubles have you brought upon yourself because of your words and actions against others?

_____

_____

5. If your relationship with others is a mirror in which you can see yourself, what does your relationship with others tell you about yourself?

_____

_____

Using your answers to the all of the foregoing questions, write a description of yourself as a person.

_____

_____

_____

Reflecting on what you have discovered in this exercise, what aspects of yourself are you happy with?

_____

_____

What would you like to change?

_____

_____

Incorporating the following guidelines into your life will move you closer to "The New You"

- Keep your priorities straight
- Always do your best
- Be good and kind to yourself and others

- Always try to make a positive difference
- Care for yourself, your work, and for others
- Be honest, be proud, be happy

The Unique Me

You have many positive qualities. What is it that makes you "you?" What qualities distinguish you from other people. Think about the things that make you unique - your physical features, your personality, your character, ways you relate to people, your intellect, your spiritual nature, your wit, your charm.

Write down those **POSITIVE** qualities that identify you as "you." Don't stop until you have listed at least thirty - list more, if you like. This may seem hard at first, but you'll be surprised at all the wonderful qualities you possess.

_____   _____
_____   _____
_____   _____
_____   _____
_____   _____
_____   _____
_____   _____
_____   _____
_____   _____
_____   _____
_____   _____
_____   _____
_____   _____
_____   _____
_____   _____

Consider which of these qualities will you still have when you have reached your weight goal?

*Your answer should be - **ALL OF THEM**

Who Am I

On ten index cards or ten pieces of paper, write thoughts or answers to the question "**Who Am I?**" Write one answer only on each card or piece of paper. When you are finished, arrange them in order of importance and write them in the spaces below.

I AM _____

I AM _____

I AM _____

I AM _____

I AM _____

I AM _____

I AM _____

I AM _____

I AM _____

I AM _____

Analyze your answers. Who are you? If your name is not at the top of the list, where are you placing yourself and your needs in relation to the other people in your life.

Write a short description about who you **WILL BE** after you reach your weight goal. Include how you will physically look, how you will feel about yourself mentally and emotionally, how you will present yourself to your family, friends, co-workers and strangers.

_____

_____

_____

_____

_____

_____

Self Drawing - Part 2

This exercise may be difficult for you for several reasons. You may not want to acknowledge how you really look or you may be so disgusted about how you look that you don't want to have to look at yourself. If you have been hiding behind your weight, it's time for you to take a realistic look at yourself. Being real with, and about yourself, is a positive step toward becoming mentally, emotionally and physically, the person you desire to be.

Compare your "*Self Drawing - Part 1*" (in the previous section) with your reflection in a full-length mirror. Compare the size, shape and proportions in the drawing to what you see in the mirror.

Is your picture an accurate representation of how you look?   YES ___ NO ___

Are you happy with your body?   YES ___ NO ___

What parts of your body do you like the most? _____

The least? _____

Did you draw any parts of your body larger than they really are?   YES ___ NO ___

If YES, which ones? _____

Why do you think you drew them larger? _____

_____

Are they parts of your body that you like or dislike? _____

Did you omit any parts of your body?   YES ___ NO ___

If yes, which ones? _____

Why do you think you left them out? _____

Are you really seeing yourself as others see you?   YES ___ NO ___

Evaluate your drawing as if it represents someone else. What does it tell you about the person who drew it?

_____

_____

Show your drawing to a friend or relative and ask them if it accurately represents your body. You might be surprised at the answers.

The New You

Write a description of what being thin means to you.

_____

_____

_____

Write a detailed description of how you will look, feel, think, act, and react once you have reached your weight goal.

_____

_____

_____

How is it different from the way you are now? _____

_____

Choose a time and location where you can be undisturbed for at least 20 minutes. If possible have your CD player within easy reach so you can pause it when instructed to do so during the exercise.

Listen to CD II – Track 3 and mentally ask yourself the following questions when instructed to do so. **Trust the first answer that comes into your mind** and write it in the space provided.

Mental Exercise 9

Mentally project yourself to a time in the future when your ideal body is your reality. You have been very successful in your efforts to achieve your weight goal, and your efforts and results have not gone unnoticed.

Imagine you are being interviewed for a feature article in a popular women's magazine. The reporter is asking you the following questions.

1. What made you decide to change your appearance and your life? _____

_____

2. Looking back over the past few weeks and months, was it difficult for you to make the changes that enabled you to reach your goal?   YES ___   NO ___

3. What adjustments did you make that helped you achieve your goal? _____

_____

4. Were the efforts you made worth it?   YES ___   NO ___

5. What was the biggest obstacle you had to overcome? _____

_____

6. How has your life changed as a result of the "Body Esteem" program? _____

_____

7. Is anyone being hurt because of your new attitude toward your appearance and your health?

YES ___   NO ___   If yes, who and how? _____

8. How are you handling their feelings? _____

_____

9. What advice would you give someone who has just made the commitment to becoming slim?

_____

_____

Turn your CD player back on and relax as you listen to the suggestions that will assist you in reaching your weight goal.

Think and act as if you have already
accomplished your goal and
it will soon be your reality

Wrap-Up

CONGRATULATIONS. YOU HAVE JUST COMPLETED "LOOKING FORWARD, THE NEW YOU." Weigh yourself and chart your progress.

This section was all about the person you are, and the person you are in the process of becoming - "The New You."

Many people have trouble recognizing and acknowledging their positive qualities. It's easier for us to beat ourselves up by focusing on what we perceive to be the negatives in our looks and personalities, especially if our self-esteem needs recharging.

If you had trouble listing positive qualities for "*The Unique Me*" exercise, show this exercise to a friend and ask them to make a list of the positive qualities they see in you. Remember – we seldom see ourselves as others see us. It's always good to get a second opinion, since we have a tendency to be too hard on ourselves. If you brush this aside, you may never know about those wonderful things that everyone else sees in you. Do this for yourself. You will probably be amazed at how other people see you and it will boost your self-esteem.

Who Are You? Are you your job? Are you somebody's mother? Are you somebody's wife? Are you still your parent's child? Initially, where did you place your name on the list? If you were already The New You would you have placed your name at the top of the list? You deserve to place yourself at the top of the list now, regardless of how many pounds overweight you are or how many demands other people place upon you.

The better you feel about yourself, the better you will be for others in your life

Start to love your body – just the way it is – right now, today. Love every part of it. The sooner you can change your attitude toward your body the sooner your body will change for you. As you learn to see yourself through kinder, less critical eyes, shame and self-hatred will melt away (and so will your excess weight). Every time you say something negative about your appearance change it into a positive statement of love and acceptance.

Begin to imagine you already have your ideal body. If you have difficulty getting a clear picture in your mind take a picture of yourself and with a marking pen draw in your ideal body on top of it, or take a picture of a body that represents your ideal body and place your face on it. What you imagine in your mind will soon become your reality.

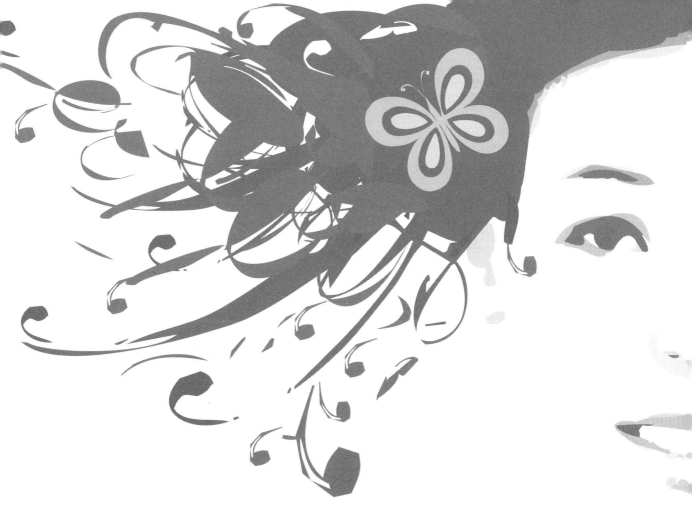

Forever Slim

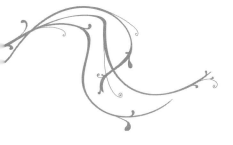

Forever Slim

Continue your success for a lifetime!

Much of this portion of your journey will have you looking back over the past weeks and comparing where you were then to where you are now. These comparisons allow you to see how far you have come and the areas where you may need to put in a little extra effort. This is also an excellent time to renew your commitment to achieving your goal.

There is no rule that says you can't go back and re-do any of the written or mental exercises in this workbook. By all means, you absolutely should go back and see if you can uncover information that may be buried deeper. Because you are more familiar with the process and less apprehensive about whether you can handle what you may encounter, you may find more experiences, feelings and emotions that you can release that will help insure your future is a slim, healthy and happy one.

This program would not be complete without addressing the issue of "Stress." Stress develops when the demands in your life exceed your ability to cope with them and your reaction to a specific stressor is different from anyone else's. While a certain level of stress is necessary to avoid boredom, high levels of stress over a sustained period can damage your health and affect your mental stability. Constant stress can suppress your immune system and make your stomach ache. Just watching a few minutes of the evening news can make your stress level soar.

Because stress is a major player in your life and it affects your health as well as your appearance, this program includes some basic information about stress and an exercise to help you identify the stressors in your life. The "*Eliminating Stress*" recording will help you control your reactions to those stressors when you encounter them.

As you reduce the intensity of your emotional and physical reactions to stress your health and your mental outlook will improve. You may even find your need to overeat or snack between meals decreasing. At the very least, you will deal with life in a more relaxed and positive way.

Continue to listen to "*The New You*" recording alternating with "*Eliminating Stress*" while you are working through this section. You may listen to any of the previous recordings as you go to sleep at night.

Food Responsiveness - 2

Check the answer that best completes the statement.

I often eat when I am not really hungry.   YES ___   NO ___

I think I am a compulsive eater.   YES ___   NO ___

I feel guilty after I overeat.   YES ___   NO ___

I feel guilty if I skip a meal.   YES ___   NO ___

I feel proud I am incorporating healthy foods into my meals.   YES ___   NO ___

Check all the statements that apply to you:

Thinking about my favorite food
___ Causes me to feel hungry
___ Makes my mouth water
___ Causes me to go to the refrigerator to get something to eat
___ Has no effect upon me
___ Has changed from an unhealthy food to a new healthy favorite!

Seeing food
___ Causes me to feel hungry
___ Makes my mouth water
___ Causes me to go to the refrigerator to get something to eat
___ Has no effect upon me

Smelling food
___ Causes me to feel hungry
___ Makes my mouth water
___ Causes me to go to the refrigerator to get something to eat
___ Has no effect upon me

Watching others eat
___ Causes me to feel hungry
___ Makes my mouth water
___ Causes me to go to the refrigerator to get something to eat
___ Has no effect upon me

I respond to food commercials on television by

    ___ Going to the refrigerator to get something to eat

    ___ Turning them off

    ___ Buying the food they are advertising

    ___ Ignoring them

    ___ Feeling disgust for the lack of integrity large commercial manufacturers show

    ___ Laughing at the ridiculous lengths commercials go to trying to sell me that junk

If I take a bite of cake, a cookie, ice cream or candy

    ___ I can't stop until I have eaten it all

    ___ I am able to take one bite and stop

    ___ I make up excuses so I won't feel guilty for eating it all

    ___ I am unaware that I am eating it all until it is gone

    ___ The question is moot . . . I am done with putting junk in my body

I experience cravings for food

    ___ When I first wake up

    ___ 1 Hour after waking up

    ___ Within 30 minutes after eating a meal

    ___ Just before bedtime

    ___ When I watch television

    ___ When I am lonely

    ___ When I am depressed

    ___ When the weather is dreary

    ___ Never

    ___ I find myself craving food, but it's wholesome, healthy food

The last time I said "NO" to a high calorie dessert was _____

I made healthy choices _____ times in the last week

Check the statement which best describes how you feel about food

    ___ I eat to live

    ___ I live to eat

Compare your answers ABOVE to the answers you wrote on "*Food Responsiveness - 1*" (Page 73).

Are any of the answers different?   YES ___   NO ___

Are your reactions to food changing?   YES ___   NO ___

Are you more aware of your reactions to food than when you started this program?   YES ___   NO ___

Guidelines for Success Revisited

Check the following Guidelines you have incorporated into your lifestyle.

___ I cleaned my closet
___ I buy form fitting clothes
___ I take pictures of my progress
___ I set reasonable and realistic goals
___ I eat regularly and don't skip meals
___ I wait when I have a craving
___ I eat slowly
___ I take the time to smell my food
___ I eat only when I am sitting down
___ I leave some food on my plate
___ I have tuned into my body
___ I eat only foods I have prepared
___ I eat everything off a plate rather than blind munching
___ I am eating from smaller plates
___ I plan meals for a week
___ I don't shop on an empty stomach
___ I shop with a list
___ I write my weight goal at the top of my grocery list
___ I buy only foods that will help me achieve my goal
___ I discuss food only at the table
___ I avoid "all you can eat" restaurants
___ I am learning about nutrition
___ I have learned to recognize emotional hunger
___ I only eat when I am physically hungry
___ I take it "one day at a time"
___ When a food commercial comes on TV I _____
___ If I blow it I _____
___ I reward myself
___ I keep busy so I don't get bored
___ I have a support system
___ I have learned to say "NO"
___ I am eating healthy

Is there anything stopping you from making all of the "Guidelines For Success" a part of your life NOW?

Recognizing Stress

If you are thinking stress is something that makes you worry, you have the wrong idea of stress. Stress is when you are worried about the things that can affect your lifestyle and includes happy things, sad things, allergic things, and physical things. Anything that causes a change in your life, even imagined change, can cause stress. Good or bad, if it's a change in your life, it's stress as far as your body is concerned and it can have both positive and negative effects on your health.

While a certain level of stress is necessary to avoid boredom, high levels of stress over a sustained period can damage your health. As a negative influence, it can result in feelings of distrust, rejection, anger, and depression, which in turn can lead to health problems such as headaches, upset stomach, rashes, insomnia, ulcers, diabetes, high blood pressure, heart disease, and stroke. And if these weren't enough reasons for you to learn to recognize and control your reactions to stress, it can also affect your weight and your ability to lose your excess weight.

Researchers from Yale University uncovered a link between the stress hormone cortisol and abdominal fat in otherwise slender women. Cortisol is an adrenal stress hormone and is an essential fight-or-flight hormone released when your body is under stress. One of the main functions of cortisol is to increase the flow of glucose, protein and fat out of your tissues and into circulation which increases your energy levels in response to a physical threat. Under normal circumstances it does its job and then allows the system to return to normal, but when you're under constant stress you can suffer from continuous elevated levels of the hormone, which can cause you to crave fats and carbohydrates. In the Yale study, published in the September/October 2000 issue of *Psychosomatic Medicine*, women with abdominal fat had exaggerated responses to cortisol. "We also found that women with greater abdominal fat had more negative moods and higher levels of life stress," said Elissa S. Epel, Ph.D., lead investigator on the study. "Greater exposure to life stress or psychological vulnerability to stress may explain their enhanced cortisol reactivity. In turn, their cortisol exposure may have led them to accumulate greater abdominal fat." Thus, recognizing and controlling your responses to the stressful situations in your life can improve your health as well as your appearance.

Following is a list of a few stress producing events. Check any of the following you have experienced in the last year:

___ Marriage	___ Divorce	___ Death of a Spouse
___ Pregnancy	___ Marital Separation	___ Marital Reconciliation
___ Death of a Relative	___ Death of a Friend	___ Change in Finances
___ Change in Residence	___ Menopause	___ Foreclosure
___ Sex Difficulties	___ Fired from Job	___ Mortgage or Loan
___ Vacation	___ Sleep less than 8 hrs.	___ Trouble with Children
___ Accident or Illness	___ Retirement	___ Trouble with In-laws
___ Traffic Jams	___ Low Calorie Diet	___ Excessive worry

Other than the forgoing, list any recurring situations that are producing stress in your life.

_____

_____

Could you change any of the above situations so they would be less stressful for you?   YES ___   NO ___

If YES, which ones? How could you change them? _____

_____

Check any of the following that are your typical reactions to stress:

___ Rapid Pulse		___ Elevated Blood Pressure	
___ Rapid Breathing		___ Feeling Light Headed	
___ Tense Muscles		___ Feeling Overwhelmed	
___ Headache		___ Lack of Emotional Control	
___ Nervousness		___ Inability to Concentrate	
___ Eating		___ Decrease in Productivity	
___ Upset Stomach		___ Lack of Motivation	
___ Loss of Memory		___ Insomnia	
___ Loss of Appetite		___ Other _____	

Are your reactions appropriate?   YES ___   NO ___

If NO, which ones are inappropriate? How could you change them? _____

_____

If you were to put your needs first in the recurring stressful situations, how would your responses change?

_____

If you possessed confidence and self assurance in the above situations would they still produce a stress response?   YES ___   NO ___

If NO, which ones would change? _____

How would your reactions to the situation change? _____

_____

How are these stresses affecting your eating habits and your weight? _____
_____

Do the situations you have listed cause you to experience the negative emotions of anger, resentment, frustration or hate?   YES ___ NO ___

Do you need stress in your life to force you to complete projects?   YES ___ NO ___ SOMETIMES ___

Do you produce stress to avoid facing a situation in your life you would rather not look at?
YES ___ NO ___
If yes, what would happen if you confronted the situation? _____
_____

List some physical and mental activities you could engage in that would help you release the stress and the tension. Examples: Take a walk, workout at a gym, meditate, listen to the *"Eliminating Stress"* program, CD II - Track 2.

_____
_____

Maintenance Tips

When you have achieved your desired goal, it's important for you to continue to exercise at least three times a week and to continue to reinforce the eating habits you have worked so hard to establish. If you slip back into your old habits, you will surely find yourself back where you were when you started this program. You really don't want that to happen, do you?

Focus on Progress – Not Perfection

Continue to weigh yourself once a week and if you find you have gained a couple of pounds immediately go back on the program outlined in "*Taking Action*" until you are back at your goal weight. It's important for you to get right back into it because the further you get away from your goal weight, the harder it is to get back on the program. Catch those two or three pounds before they become twenty. Don't make excuses - **DO IT NOW**.

When you are once again back at your goal weight, give yourself another week to stabilize by reviewing and following the program in "*Self-Reflections & Self-Love*". Be sure you continue to exercise every day. Try to determine the amount and types of food that will allow you to eat a balanced diet without gaining weight.

Following are a few tips to help you maintain your goal weight. Some of these ideas may already be a part of your lifestyle, while others may need to be incorporated to ensure your continued success.

Breathe Stress Away

If you do feel stressed in a situation, take a few slow deep breaths and as you slowly exhale, mentally remind yourself to relax. Gently redirect your thoughts away from whatever is causing the stress and redirect your thoughts to your breathing. Focus on each breath until you feel calm and relaxed. (You can do this in heavy traffic when you are running late or even in a heated discussion.)

Find the subtle beauty in the world around you. Be thankful for the rare and precious gift of life itself.

Drink More Water

Drinking water hydrates, cleanses and helps balance your system.

Eat "Raw" Foods

Raw foods are higher in nutritional value when all of the nutrients have not been lost by over cooking. Choose green salads in place of pasta, and fresh fruit instead of pastries for dessert.

Nutrition First

Eating foods that contain the highest nutritional value first will insure you are satisfying your nutritional requirements before you fill up on foods containing a higher calorie content. Your stomach also digests what it gets first more efficiently.

Always Look For Ways to Improve the Quality of the Food You Eat

Start changing your eating habits to include vegan meals at least one day a week. If you take the time and care to prepare attractive and nutritious meals, you'll probably find you are doing it two or three times a week. You will be consuming fewer calories and less fat as you develop a healthier way of eating. Cutting out animal products from a meal increases fiber, reduces fat and chances for an allergic reaction.

Second Helpings

They are a NO-NO, unless it's fruit or raw vegetables.

Read Labels

Purchase canned fruits packed in natural juice, avoid foods that contain added sugar or salt. Purchase tuna packed in water. If you have oil-packed tuna on hand, drain off as much oil as you can, then run some hot water over the tuna and drain. This helps to remove any excess oil, (and the extra calories).

Sweets

Of course you want them . . . but, do you really need them? If you can't say **NO**, share a dessert and limit yourself to a very small portion. A better alternative is to substitute fresh fruit for the high calorie desserts.

Snack Food

Pretzels, Potato Chips, Snack Crackers, Dips . . . easy to munch on, yet a huge source of calories and fat. Check the labels for calories and ingredients, as you should with all packaged foods you buy. Notice the **serving size** and try to limit yourself to **one** serving. You will probably find you're more satisfied by a healthy snack alternative as suggested in the "**Eating For Life**" section at the back of this book.

Eating at Someone's Home

Practice saying "It really was delicious, but I just couldn't eat another bite." Don't let anyone intimidate you into eating something you really don't want, or eating more than you really need.

Plan Ahead

If you know you have a special occasion coming up, plan ahead! Run through the event and see yourself making healthy choices. Yes, one bite of birthday cake tastes the same as eating the entire thing, so why not enjoy just a bite and leave the binging to people who are still sleep eating through life.

Wrap-Up

CONGRATULATIONS FOR COMPLETING ALL EIGHT SECTIONS OF THIS PROGRAM!
Weigh and measure yourself and chart your progress.

We know at times it has been a struggle for you and has taken a real commitment on your part. We acknowledge you for having the strength and determination to overcome the obstacles that have stood in the way of reaching your goal. You have done something good for yourself that will change the rest of your life.

This is a good time for you to compare where you were a few weeks ago and where you are now. How have your reactions to food changed, do you feel different physically, do you have more energy, do you feel healthier?

Do you have a better understanding of why you gained your weight and what it represents? Do you know how to maintain your losses in the future?

How has your self talk changed? Are your thoughts more positive? When you have a negative thought do you immediately change it to a positive one?

If you have not as yet achieved your ideal weight, continue to use the tools, techniques and recordings that are part of this program until you reach your goal. When you reach your goal, continue to monitor your weight and if you gain a couple of pounds immediately look for the reason. Has your self talk become negative, are you suppressing anger, have you slipped back into old eating patterns, are you eating for emotional reasons, are you experiencing more stress than usual, have you stopped exercising? Try to discover what has changed in your life, or your thinking, and listen to the recording that relates to that particular issue until you are back on track.

Be proud of yourself for making your health and your appearance priority in your life. You have a bright and wonderful future to look forward to.

What you conceive in your mind
and believe in your heart
you can achieve

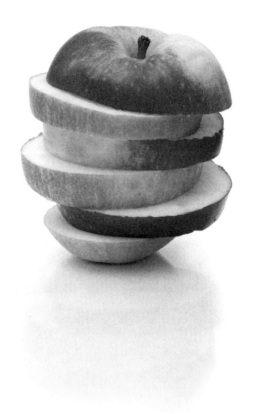

Eating For Life

Eating For Life

Food, at the most basic level, is fuel for your body. Food sustains your life force, you need it to continue to live and thrive. If you want your body to work efficiently and effectively you need to give it the best nutritional support you can.

Eating right isn't as hard as you might imagine. With a basic understanding of how different foods affect your body and mind, you'll discover that eating for health is essentially about balance and enjoying more of the food provided by nature.

We included this section to introduce you to some simple truths about food. You probably already know the basics of eating well, so we've tried to keep it short and focused on healthy eating. It's a primer to a new perspective on food, one we hope you will continue to expand through continued self-education. Our philosophy is that you are ultimately responsible for your body and what you put into it. Through self-awareness and education you can return to your natural state of health.

Don't Diet, Eat For Life

Your goal should be to eat a balanced amount of protein, carbohydrates and fats coming from high quality, nutrient rich, low calorie foods that nurture your body. By focusing on health and not deprivation, you'll be flushing the toxins that have built up in your body. Your skin will become bright and beautiful. You might even find the dark circles under your eyes have disappeared. You'll look better, feel better and most importantly, you'll develop a way of eating that will sustain your health, beauty, and slim figure for a lifetime.

Proteins

Protein contains 4 calories per gram. Protein is comprised of essential amino acids. They are called essential because your body needs them to survive. Since your body does not produce these "essential" amino acids, you must introduce them into your body through the foods you eat. Protein helps to build, maintain, and repair tissue, including muscle.

Most foods contain a number of amino acids. Meats, eggs and soy contain all nine (9) essential amino acids. There are other lesser known possibilities. Quinoa, a "super" grain, is another source of complete proteins. It is important to note, since most foods contain a number of the amino acids, if you are eating healthy, balanced meals throughout the day you will no doubt ingest all nine (9) essential amino acids.

Animal sources:	*Vegetarian sources:*
Meat	Nuts
Poultry	Seeds
Fish	Legumes
Eggs	Whole grains
Dairy Products	Some Vegetables

Meat, Poultry and Fish:

Whenever possible **choose hormone and antibiotic free, free-range meats**. Most major chains carry these meats and you can find them at health oriented markets. Also choose leaner cuts of meat. One alternative to red meats, is **Ostrich,** which has been gaining popularity because it is naturally lean.

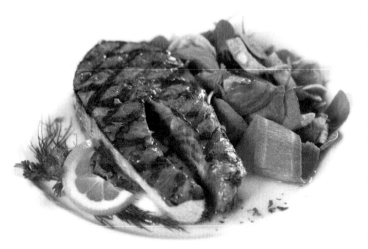

Chicken and turkey breast is an excellent source of protein. And remember, always remove the skin before cooking, since the skin is extremely fatty.

There is a wonderful variety of fish in the oceans and rivers of this bountiful world. Many health professionals advise at least two servings a week of cold water fish that are high in Omega-3 fatty acids (a.k.a. "Good Fats"), such as salmon, haddock, cod, tuna, mahi mahi, tilapia, halibut, mackerel and sardines. **Try to buy wild caught fish, rather than "farm raised." Wild fish is generally tastier, leaner and healthier for you.**

Dairy:

Rich in calcium, dairy products eaten in moderation, can be a healthy addition to most diets. Some people, however, are allergic to dairy or are lactose intolerant and should incorporate dairy substitutes into their diet. Since dairy products can be high in saturated fats, it's best to choose low-fat dairy products such as low-fat milk, low-fat plain yogurt (mix in your favorite fruit or sweetener, such as agave and alcohol-free vanilla), and low-fat cottage cheese and hard cheese. **Try to choose organic, hormone-free dairy products whenever possible.**

Soy:

Soy products have gained incredible popularity. It's ability to be manipulated to resemble other foods such as "soy chicken" and "soy milk" makes it seem like the perfect alternative for the vegetarians. Some studies of soy indicate it may protect against heart disease and reduce the risk of breast cancer. Howerver, other studies have shown a number of dangers associated with soy products, ranging from the depression of thyroid function to increased risk of digestive related cancer. You can learn for yourself about this highly controversial plant by doing a little research in your local library or on the web. Learn more at www.soyonlineservice.co.nz and www.westonaprice.org/soy/index.html.

Because of soy's hormonal interaction indications, it's a good idea for you to see your health professional who can evaluate your unique body chemistry and make recommendations for your specific condition and age. **If you do choose a soy based product, be sure it is organically grown, NON-GMO soy.**

Non-Animal Protein Sources:

If you are a vegetarian, vegan or simply trying to avoid animal products there is a bounty of sources provided by nature. **Raw nuts, seeds, beans, and lentils are excellent sources of concentrated protein.**

Whole grains, while normally thought of as a carbohydrate, can provide a good source of protein as well. Barley, Brown rice, Buckwheat, Millet, Oatmeal, Rye, and Wheat germ are common sources of protein. **Super grains** include Amaranth, Quinoa, Millet, Brown Rice, Pharinah, Kamut, and Spelt. We suggest **sprouted grain** cereals and breads. According to the Price-Pottenger Nutrition Foundation, sprouted grains are nutrient rich and easier to digest.

Protein Powders:

Hemp protein powder is one of the most nutritious way to add protein to your smoothie. The fatty acid profile of the hemp seed is extremely beneficial, containing omega-6 and omega-3 fatty acids in a virtually ideal ratio. Try to avoid flavored "protein powders" that are full of calories, sweeteners, and chemical additives.

Carbohydrates

As with protein, carbohydrates contain 4 calories per gram. In simple terms, carbohydrates provide fuel for your body and food for your brain. This is often a misunderstood area of healthy eating, especially when people think of "dieting."

Not eating enough carbs or eating "empty carbs" may leave you feeling tired and foggy.

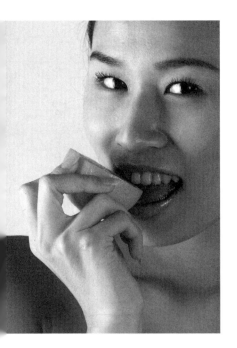

Forget about the "low carb" labeled foods and concentrate on eating the right kind of carbohydrates. Eating "smart carbs" will deliver energy to your mind and body. You'll feel great and you'll be slimming down.

Carbohydrates come in one of two forms: Complex or Simple.

Complex carbohydrates are made up of multiple nutrients, these are the "smart carbs" your body needs. They take longer to break down and digest in your body. Starches and fiber (whole foods) are examples of complex carbohydrates and tend to be low on the Glycemic Index.

Simple carbohydrates are made up of only one or two nutrients. These are the "empty carbs" that go straight to your hips and increase your risk of diabetes. Simple carbohydrates break down quickly causing your blood sugar level to rise more rapidly. When your blood sugar rises rapidly, your body releases excess amounts of insulin. Sugars, such as table sugar, tend to be processed and refined and are high on the Glycemic Index.

In general, you want most of your carbs to come from complex carbohydrates. Good sources of complex carbohydrates are whole fruits and vegetables as well as whole grains. Of course, even with smart carbs, there is always the risk of too much of a good thing. Just be sure to eat a sensible portion according with your lifestyle.

The Beauty of Whole Grains

Whole grains have not been refined and contain more nutrients (more protein, fiber, vitamins and minerals). They have not been stripped of their nutritional value or flavor. Oatmeal, brown rice, and whole wheat are examples of whole grains. They will be more

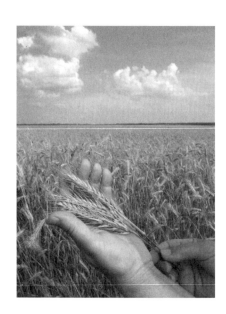

dense, coarser and chewier, and the taste will be stronger than their refined counterparts (white bread, white pasta, white rice, and foods made with white flour and white sugar).

Initially, you may not like the taste and texture of whole grains; but, if you gradually introduce them into your diet, you will come to enjoy them and prefer them to their nutritionally void counterparts.

"Spouted" grains are even a better option, according to the Price-Pottenger Nutrition Foundation of La Mesa, California, because sprouting is best way to release all of the vital nutrients stored in whole grains. An excellent company making exceptional organic spouted grain products is "Food For Life" (www.foodforlife.com).

Start by introducing whole grains into your meals along with other foods. For instance, whole grain pastas make great hearty fall and winter dishes and the whole grains will give the dish more nutritional value. Use them with your favorite marinara sauce or in soups, such as minestrone. Brown and wild rice are good with stir-fried or sautéed vegetables. You might be surprised to find that many of the new Asian style restaurants will have brown rice available upon request.

Whole grain flours are great for most baking and make great tasting pancakes. Have fun and experiment!

Whole grain porridge can be a wonderful filling breakfast. Oatmeal is the most popular of the breakfast grains. The best oatmeal to eat is the slow cooking kind. The slow cooking oatmeal is fully intact, meaning it hasn't been stripped of any of the nutrients. Quick cooking oats cook quickly because they have been stripped of their outer layer, which decreases the fiber content allowing it to cook more quickly.

Try other grain cereals including mixed grain cereals or make your own. A wonderful combination is rolled oats and rye flakes. If you would like it to be higher in protein add Quinoa and/or Amaranth, which are both high protein grains.

Tasty Toppings for grain cerals

- Fresh fruit
- Cinnamon, pumpkin pie spice, nutmeg
- Vanilla extract, almond extract
- Walnuts, pecans, or sliced almonds
- A sprinkling of dried coconut
- A splash of raw agave nectar
- A few raisins or dried cranberries

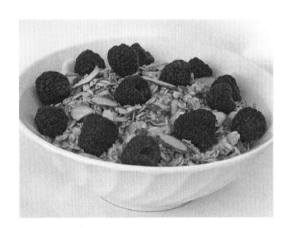

Fats

Unlike protein and carbohydrates, fats contain 9 calories per gram. A healthful diet should contain a daily caloric intake of 20-30% fats. Aside from making foods taste good, fats play an important role in any diet. They help with the digestion of food, creation of hormones, transportation of nutrients, increasing immunity to disease, and making you feel full.

Unsaturated Fats - Healthy Fats

Unsaturated fats are considered good fats. These fats have been shown to increase good cholesterol levels. The most healthful of the unsaturated fats are monounsaturated fats. Monounsaturated fats are found in avocados, olives and olive oils, canola oils, nut and seed oils. In general, unsaturated fats come from plant sources.

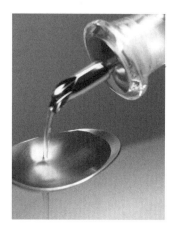

Cold-Pressed Extra Virgin Olive Oil: #1 choice for uncooked preparation such a salad dressings.

Omega 3 fatty acids are a healthful fat, which definitely should be included in a healthy diet. Good sources of this fat are flaxseeds, walnuts and cold water fish such as salmon, sardines and mackerel.

Saturated Fats

Saturated fats raise total blood cholesterol levels because they tend to boost both good HDL and bad LDL cholesterol. Animal based saturated fats (meats, dairy and lard) have been shown to be the worst. Organic Coconut and Palm Oils are a better alternative.

Trans Fatty Acids

Trans fats, or trans fatty acids, are man made saturated fats and should be avoided as much as possible. Sources of trans fatty acids are hydrogenated oils found in such foods as some margarines and vegetable shortening, which are commonly used in commercial cookies, cakes, and a host of fast foods.

The Good	The Bad	The Ugly
Organic Cold-Press Olive Oil, Nut and Seed Oils *Example:* *Olive and Flaxseed Oil*	Animal Based Fats (Meat, Dairy Products, Lard) *Example:* *Butter*	Hydrogenated Oil Products *Example:* *Shortening,* *Many Packaged Products*

Nuts about Nuts

Raw nuts and seeds are a good source of protein and dietary fiber. Nuts are high in good fats, vitamins, and fiber and can be included as a part of a healthy diet. However, nuts are also a very concentrated food so be sure to eat them in moderation. And if you don't already, stay away from cooked nuts! Raw is the way nature intended nuts to be eaten.

Why not roast nuts? Because heating nuts at higher temperatures transforms the healthy unsaturated fatty acids into a fat that acts like a saturated fatty acid. Heating also destroys the natural enzymes contained in the nut. These enzymes, such as lipase, are needed to digest the fat.

Facts About Nuts

• Nuts and seeds are the richest source of vitamin E. In fact, 1/2 cup of almonds contains over twice the daily requirement of vitamin E.

• Most nuts and seeds are high in potassium: about 4 oz of almonds, Brazil nuts, peanuts, pine nuts, pistachios, and sunflower seeds each provide more than 500 mg of potassium. Almonds, pistachio, flax, pumpkin and sesame seeds are very high in iron. A cup of almonds, Brazil nuts, filberts or pistachios, or an ounce of sesame seeds contain as much calcium as a cup of milk.

• Nuts and seeds also contain other minerals such as magnesium, phosphorus, and zinc, and are rich in vitamin B.

• Almonds are high in folic acid.

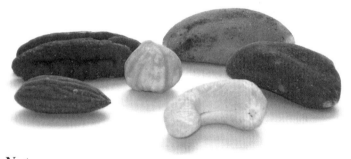

Tips for Eating Nuts

• Break a couple of walnuts or pecans over your morning oatmeal

• Instead of a candy bar for an afternoon snack, have a small hand-full of raw nuts

• Sprinkle some almonds or pine nuts over a salad

Whole Foods

Whole foods are foods that are as close to their natural states as possible, in other words unrefined and unprocessed.

The Wholesome Facts

• Whole foods also tend to be high in fiber.

• Fiber stabilizes your blood sugar and leaves you with that "full" feeling.

• Fiber also helps eliminate toxins from your body and helps with the digestion process.

• Whole fruits, vegetables, whole grains, and beans are excellent sources of fiber.

For the most part, whole foods do not affect your blood sugar levels like processed or refined foods. However, some whole foods, like bananas and carrots, may increase your blood sugar, but they are still considered to be healthful and contain necessary vitamins and minerals.

Fresh Produce Tips

• Try to eat at least five helpings of fruits and vegetables a day.

• Whenever possible buy organic, locally grown produce.

• Another great idea is to visit your local Farmers market. Farmers markets not only provide the greatest variety of fresh, locally grown seasonal produce, they also provide an assortment of other local goods such as freshly baked whole grain breads, nuts and seeds, flowers, etc. Farmers markets are a great place to take the family. Children can help pick out their favorite fruits and vegetables and sample new ones.

Processed and Refined Products: The Anti-Whole Foods

Processed and refined foods are the opposite of whole foods. The processing and refining process strips whole foods of their nutrients, i.e., the fiber, vitamins and minerals. In essence when you eat refined foods you are eating empty calories. You are eating foods that may fill your body and alleviate your hunger, but you are not providing your body with the vitamins and minerals it needs to keep you healthy.

Glycemic Index-
It's All About Balance

The American Journal of Clinical Nutrition created the Glycemic Index (GI) which ranks how quickly the body breaks down certain foods and converts them into sugar on a scale of 1 to 100. When you eat foods high on the Glycemic Index, the nutrients enter your blood stream quickly elevating your body's blood sugar causing your pancreas to release insulin. The insulin then encourages those nutrients to be deposited as fat in order to stabilize your blood sugar. Highly refined products such as sugar, white flour, white rice, and foods containing these products (i.e. pastries) receive high ratings on the GI.

According to "Glycemic Solution's" clinical research, there are basically two ways the body reacts to all food. The reaction is dependent upon the GI of the food or drink.

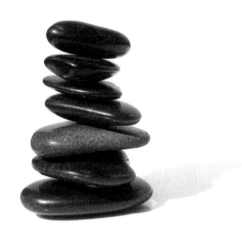

- High glycemic foods elevate blood glucose and insulin levels, and **stimulate fat-storage.**

- Low glycemic foods do not overly elevate blood glucose and insulin, and do not stimulate Lipoprotein Lipase (LPL) fat-storing mechanisms.

Since we are all different, you need to tune into your own body and become aware of your sensitivities to certain types of food and additives.

How do you feel and act after you've eaten carbohydrates that are high on the GI?
Do you feel light headed or queasy, do you become easily agitated, or do you feel shaky, tired or sleepy? How do you feel and act after you have eaten protein, fats, and whole foods low on the GI?

Following an eating plan rich in low GI foods will help you feel satisfied longer because of the slower rate of sugar absorption into the blood. This also means your energy levels are more consistent throughout the day.

In general, eating a balanced amount of high quality proteins, carbohydrates and fats periodically through the day will keep your blood sugar stable and your energy high. An important factor to consider when choosing foods is the fiber content. High fiber foods work in conjunction with the GI of a food to deliver a lower overall "Glycemic Load." Learn more at www.glycemicindex.com.

By maintaining a balanced GI level, not only will you lose weight faster, you are helping to reduce your chance of developing diabetes, heart disease and cancer!

The Sweet Life

No nutrition section would be complete without a note on sweets. After all, not only do sweets taste good they are an integral part of our social system. Who would want Thanksgiving without pumpkin or pecan pie or a birthday without a birthday cake?

Traditional sweets/desserts are usually high on the glycemic index, high in saturated fats, and high in calories. And of course they have . . . sugar. Gary Null, Ph.D., a well regarded authority on healthy living, says, "High up on my list of things that cause cells to be attacked, cause disease, and cause premature aging is this white poison (and sugar substitutes as well)."

A study, published in the *American Journal of Clinical Nutrition* (November, 2006) from Karolinska Institute showed a direct link between the high consumption of sugar sweetened food and beverages and an increased risk of developing pancreatic cancer. In fact, sugar has been linked to numerous health dangers including contributing to type 2 diabetes, obesity, heart disease, improper bowel function, risk of breast cancer . . . and the list goes on. Unfortunately, if current habits continue for Americans, one out of every three women in the U.S. will develop diabetes.

THE USUAL SUSPECTS - Dangerous Sweeteners
The following is a list of the usual low-cost, extremely unhealthy ingredients popular in commercial junk food. It's better just to think of these unnatural ingredients as poison if you are serious about improving your health:

- **Corn syrup**
- **High fructose corn syrup**
- **Refined white (table) sugar**
- **Artificial sweeteners such as aspartame**

Rule #1: A little goes a long way. One bite of cake tastes the same as eating the whole cake.

Rule #2: Eating healthy is not depriving yourself, it's <u>finding better options</u>.

AGAVE NECTAR is one of the very best sweeteners! This gift from nature has a low glycimic index and is extremely sweet. Agave nectar works great as a honey and maple syrup substitute for people who need to avoid high glycemic foods. It's also great for cooking since it doesn't crystallize.

Experiment with different types of more healthful sweeteners such as **evaporated cane juice, fruit sweeteners, Sucanant, Rapadura, honey, brown rice syrup, and barley malt syrup.**

Some people have the tendency to suddenly think that because they are eating a more healthful slice of pie, that they can suddenly indulge in more than they would have before. Remember, calories are calories, you still need to be mindful. Even though your new sweets might be healthier, treat them with the same discretion you would any sweets and eat them in moderation.

Shhhhh...here's the secret weapon for your sweet tooth . . . STEVIA!!!

What's that . . . you haven't heard of the zero calorie 100% natural sweetener that won't rot your teeth and comes from the leaves of a plant found in the rain forests of South America? Well, that's the way the multi-billion dollar sugar and the artificial sweetener industry would like to keep it.

What you may not know is Stevia is already incredibly popular in other parts of the world, most notably, Japan. Stevia accounts for nearly 40% of the Japanese sweetener market. Because of its use in Japan, there is much more scientific evidence of Stevia's safety than for most foods and additives. These extensive studies have found Stevia to be safe with no side effects. In 2006, The World Health Organization (WHO) performed a thorough evaluation of recent experimental studies of stevioside and steviols conducted on animals and humans concluding that it was perfectly safe as a food additive and might even be shown to have some positive effects on hypertension and type-2 diabetes. But unlike other popular "patented" zero calorie sweeteners allowed by the FDA that have numerous reported serious side effects and have made corporations rich for no justifiable reason, the FDA continues to inexplicably label Stevia as a "dietary supplement." For that reason, you will not find Stevia in commercial food products.

What began as a product in the back of health food stores has started to appear in more main stream stores. If you can't find it in your local store, ask them to carry it, and in the meantime you can order it on-line on most popular health food web sites and amazon.com. You can even grow the plant, "Stevia rebaudiana," yourself (check out www.stevia.net for tips). With your own plants you can enjoy the dried leaves in a powdered form or extract leaves into a liquid yourself. Unprocessed Stevia is 30 times sweeter than sugar!

Stevia has NO CALORIES and NO AFFECT ON BLOOD SUGAR, yet once processed, is 100 to 300 times sweeter than sugar. It may take a little transition time to learn the right amount to use, but after awhile you might wonder how you ever got along without it.

It comes most commonly in the both a powder and liquid. We personally like the alcohol free liquid form of Stevia for beverages and smoothies. You can even find flavored versions of liquid Stevia, such as vanilla, chocolate and lemon. The best powdered form of Stevia, such as *Stevia Plus* from Sweetleaf, uses inulin fiber. People use Stevia as a sugar substitute in everything from baked apple crisp to sweet iced green tea. You can find plenty of information to help you integrate Stevia into your new healthy lifestyle in several wonderful books and websites. Learn more at www.stevia.net.

Real Chocolate Bliss

Known as the "Food of the Goddesses," chocolate holds a special place in the hearts of most women. Most women have not yet learned to enjoy real chocolate. In fact, many of the things we label as chocolate actually have very little chocolate. The primary ingredient in most chocolate bars, chocolate syrup, chocolate ice cream, is not chocolate, but instead, processed sugar or high-fructose corn syrup. When the experts explain the beneficial effects of chocolate, they are referring to the real deal . . . the darker, the better.

Real chocolate, also known in nature as "cacao," is an extraordinary super food rich in antioxidants. Cacao actually contains very little natural sugar and is bitter. Sweeteners are used to balance the bitterness of the chocolate. You can now find raw cacao in it's natural form (the cacao bean) and powder form.

Since you now have some wonderful alternatives to processed sweeteners, you can enjoy your very own guilt-free chocolate indulgences. An excellent place to expand your knowledge about chocolate, along with some amazing "raw" recipes, can be found in the book, *Naked Chocolate*, by David Wolf and Shazzie (www.naked-chocolate.com).

Water and Other Healthful Drinks

Try to drink at least 64 oz of water a day. This can be difficult, but there are many ways to achieve this goal. Start by keeping a sport bottle of water with you at all times. This will help you gauge your input during the day.

Since 74% of the body is made up of water, you'll want to drink only the purest water possible. While municipalities attempt to provide "safe" drinking water, normal tap water still contains a number of harmful substances. The first danger is Chlorine. Used as a disinfectant, Chlorine has been associated with atherosclerosis (hardening and narrowing of the arteries) and cancer. Other substances in tap water may include microorganisms which the chlorine is unable to kill. Finally, tap water may contain industrial pollutants, drug residues, fluoride, organic chemicals, and toxic minerals and metals.

- Drink water first thing in the morning.

- Keep water in your car and with you at work.

- At home, drink water from your favorite glass.

- Try to drink **only filtered water or bottled spring water**.

- Start a water club at work. Many well know bottled water companies deliver. Splitting the cost between 5-6 people (or as many as would like to join) makes the price very reasonable.

Juice Tips

- If you do choose fruit juice, try make your own juice and drink it immediately. This will ensure you receive the greatest benefit from the fresh juice.

- Try juicing fresh fruits and vegetables. Experiment with combinations like apple/celery.

- **Avoid** fruit juice sweetened with sugar, fructose, high fructose corn syrup and any chemical/artificial sweeteners.

- If you do enjoy the taste of fruit juice but want to limit your intake, cut it with some mineral water.

- Try mineral water with a splash of cranberry juice in a champagne glass.

- Add fresh seasonal fruit to fresh filtered water, mineral water or homemade caffeine-free ice tea.

- Adding mint and/or a cucumber slice to water also makes a wonderfully delicious drink.

- Freeze your favorite fruit juice in ice cube trays and use them for ice in water.

Read Labels!!! We can't emphasize this enough. Get into the habit of reading the labels on everything you buy or want to buy. "Ok," you say, "But what does all that information mean?" Below are guidelines to follow when reading labels.

Old Fashioned Oats

① ② ③ ④ ⑤

Nutrition Facts

Serving Size: 1/2 cup dry (40g)

Amount Per Serving	As Served
Calories 150	**Calories from Fat** 25

	% Daily Value
Total Fat 3g	4%
Saturated Fat 0.5g	2%
Cholesterol 0g	0%
Sodium 0g	2%
Total Carbohydrate 27g	9%
Dietary Fiber 4g	15%
Sugars 1g	
Protein 0g	

Vitamin A 0%	•	Vitamin C 0%
Calcium 0%	•	Iron 10%

Percent Daily Values are based on a 2,000 calorie diet. Your daily values may be higher or lower depending on your calorie needs:

	Calories	2,000	2,500
Total Fat	Less than	65g	80g
Sat Fat	Less than	20g	80g
Cholesterol	Less than	300mg	300mg
Sodium	Less than	2,400mg	2,400mg
Total Carbohydrate		300g	375g
Dietary Fiber		25g	30g

⑥ **Ingredients:** Rolled Oats

① *Check the serving size.*
Many packages contain more than one serving. How much do you actually eat versus the serving size? **You may think you are eating one serving, when in fact you are eating 2 or 3 servings.**

② *Read the calories per serving.*

③ *Check the fat, carbohydrates, protein and sodium.*
What is the percent of fat from saturated fat versus unsaturated fat? Many low-fat or low-sugar items contain more sodium than their counterparts.
Pay careful attention to the grams of **dietary fiber (more is the better) and **sugar** (as little as possible).

④ *Read the Nutritional Values*
This lists the percent of the daily recommended vitamins and minerals for the average person.

⑤ *Understand Daily Values*
These recommendations are examples for consumers. **Your target calories and fat-gram daily totals are probably lower than what is listed on most labels (as prescribed by your doctor or nutritionist).**

⑥ *Read the ingredients listed on the label.*
Ingredients are listed from largest to smallest amount by weight. This means what is inside the package, can, or jar contains the largest amount of the first ingredient and the smallest amount of the last ingredient.

If the list does not fit on the label or there are ingredients you do not recognize or cannot pronounce—these are indications that this is a food product and not a whole food.

Use the ingredient list to spot things you'd like to avoid, such as palm oil, which is high in saturated fat. Also try to avoid hydrogenated oils that are high in trans fat. They are not listed by total amount on the label, but you can choose foods that don't list *hydrogenated or partially hydrogenated oil* in the ingredient list.

At the Supermarket

Become familiar with your local health food market. These stores are popping up all over because more people are realizing the benefits of eating healthy. They offer fresh, organic fruits and vegetables, hormone and antibiotic free meats, vitamins and minerals, and dairy alternatives, just to name a few. Many of these stores also offer classes designed to teach you more about healthy foods, and their benefits.

The following will help you stay on track when you are shopping:

- #1 ALWAYS READ THE NUTRITIONAL INFORMATION AND INGREDIENTS ON THE LABEL OF EVERY PACKAGED FOOD YOU CONSIDER PURCHASING

- Don't shop when you are hungry

- Create a meal plan for the week and then **shop with a list**

- Beware of "mini-snacks"—tiny crackers, cookies and pretzels. Most people end up eating more than they realize, and the calories add up

- Choose foods packaged in individual serving sizes

- If organic produce is too expensive for your budget, buy non-organic and wash the fruits and vegetables well. Most important is that you eat as much fresh produce as possible.

Meal Replacement Product Technology

Meal replacement bars, powders and drinks have become a lucrative area for the diet industry. In truth, nothing can replace the health benefits of wholesome fresh foods. Yet, in our busy lives, these options can sound quite appealing. The problem with these highly processed products is that they are usually far from natural. They are the result of food engineers in a lab who are far more concerned about developing a product that can sit on shelves for years and still be addictive.

Not much better than a candy bar, these products are often full of some of the worst ingredients, including high fructose corn syrup, chemical flavoring and a host of preservatives. In fact, your body has to work very little to break down the compounds in these products.

The processed sugars packed into these products are definitely not good for your health or your waistline. You might be horrified by the amount of sugar they pack into these bars.

Even the "healthy" bars are quite often high in sugars, as they are often meant to act as an "energy" bar. That's great if you're in the middle of a triathlon, but not so helpful if you are simply doing a half hour work out . . . or even worse, not doing anything active at all to burn the calories.

Always read the nutritional information and ingredients on the package before purchasing.

At Home

Whenever possible plan and prepare your own meals. Begin to get in touch with the enjoyment you can receive from it's preparation - cutting up the vegetables, the scent/fragrance of the chicken marinade, the feeling of slicing a fresh apple. Make as many meals as possible an enjoyable experience and not just a chore or a "have to" activity.

After you have prepared the meal, sit down and enjoy it, turn off the TV, don't answer the phone, eat at the dinning room table with the entire family. Let meals be a time to reconnect with yourself and your family.

These hints may help you achieve your goal:

- Eat a substantial breakfast and lunch, while making dinner the lightest meal, rather than the heaviest meal.

- Eat your dinner at least three hours before bedtime.

- Use smaller plates at meals.

- Serve food in the appropriate portion amounts and don't go back for seconds.

- Put away any leftovers in separate, portion-controlled amounts. Consider freezing the portions you likely won't eat for a while.

- Never eat out of the bag or carton.

- Don't keep platters of food on the table. You will be more likely to "pick" at it or have a second serving without realizing it.

- Don't eat off someone else's plate, especially your children's. You won't need to clean their plate for them if you judge the serving sizes accurately. If there are foods they have never tried or don't like, give them a very small portion.

- **Dressing For Success**: Commercial salad dressings can be full of trans fats, additives and preservatives so be sure to read those labels to find a healthy dressing. Why not make your own? Olive oil and balsamic vinegar makes a very tasty dressing and you can spice it up with your favorite mustard, soy sauce, or agave nectar. Fresh lemon juice and olive oil is another wonderful dressing.

Eating Out

One of life's greatest joys is eating out with friends and family; however, it can pose a challenge for ordering/eating healthy. Many restaurants have increased their portions to unhealthy sizes and use an unhealthy amount of saturated fat and salt.

The following tips may help you successfully navigate the restaurant experience:

- Begin by filtering the menu. Find the healthiest meals and choose from those choices. Eventually, this will become habit.

- Speak Up! Don't be afraid to ask how the food is prepared and make sure you are getting what you want. Restaurants often have alternatives such as wheat bread rather than white bread for sandwiches.

- Ask to have olive oil used when preparing the meal instead of butter.

- Ask for half or smaller portions.

- Split a meal with someone and order a small side salad.

- Order a cup of broth based soup and a healthy appetizer, or a salad instead of a full meal.

- Ask to have a salad, fresh fruit, or steamed veggies substituted for the usual side dishes that accompany an entree, such as fries or mashed potatoes.

- Bring your own salad dressing or order it on the side—opt for the oil-based dressings instead of cream based dressings (remember the oil-based dressings often contain good fat).

- For protein, try opting for fish or chicken. Choose entrées without cream sauces and are baked, broiled or steamed. Avoid fried foods.

- Eyeball your appropriate portion, set the rest aside, and ask for a "to go" box right away. Servings at many American restaurants are often big enough to provide lunch for two days.

- Try not to eat the white flour bread many restaurants automatically give you at the beginning of a meal. White bread and tortilla chips are just empty calories that can easily undermine all your good eating that day. If everyone agrees, ask that they remove it.

- Order imported sparkling water at a fine restaurant for an guilt-free indulgence instead of soda or alcohol.

Deceptive "To Go" Drinks

- **Smoothies:** These can seem like a healthy choice in lieu of the typical fast food meal, but do be careful. Most of these drinks pack in a lot of calories and many contain an obscene amount of sugar.

  For example, a 24 Ounce "Banana Berry" smoothie from Jamba Juice contains a whopping 480 calories. Those calories are from the <u>99 grams of sugar</u>, with only 4 grams of fiber and 5 grams of protein.

  That little smoothie that is supposed to be so healthy and full of energy is going to spike your insulin levels and goes straight to your hips . . . unless of course you plan to be running a marathon that day.

  The bottom line is **<u>before you order any smoothies, find out the ingredients and nutritional content</u>**. Try to avoid smoothies made with sorbet and juices from concentrate. Smoothies are usually made in a "juice bar," so a better alternative might be a small glass of fresh juice.

- **Coffee Drinks:** Caffeine-free tea is always a better alternative, but if you love your coffee experience . . . beware of the flavored drinks. These drinks are full of sugar, artificial flavors, and more sugar. In a venti "Mochacino Maddness" and "Caramel Triple Calorie Latte" you're likely to find almost half your calories for the entire day in one cup! Try to keep it simple and small, such as an unsweetened non-fat latte.

  Fact #1: Designer coffee drinks are full of sugar. While a 16 oz. non-fat latte has 160 calories, the same size non-fat "White Chocolate Mocha" (without the whipped cream) from Starbucks contains 340 calories.

  Fact #2: Green tea drinks aren't always good for you. A Starbucks 16 oz. "Blackberry Green Tea Frappuccino® Blended Crème (without the whipped cream on top) has 430 calories and 73 grams of sugar!

  Fact #3: "Light" drinks use the term loosely. Take for example, a 16 oz. "Banana Coconut Frappuccino® Light Blended Coffee - no whip" from Starbucks has 310 calories and 55 grams of sugar.

Learn about the ingredients and caloric content of your favorite drinks by visiting their web sites:

Jamba Juice: www.jambajuice.com/menuguide/index.html
Starbucks Coffee: www.starbucks.com/retail/nutrition_info.asp

Further Reading

Our focus in this workbook has been to empower you with self-knowledge so you can break free from the negative thoughts that have literally weighed you down. Chances are you're well on your way to eating for health after taking the Body Esteem journey. But just in case you'd like more inspiration or guidance on the path to healthy eating, we encourage you to check out our web site at **www.bodyesteem.com** for recipes, articles and contributions posted from your sisters on the journey.

In addition to the web sites previously listed in this book, we recommend the following web sites to assist you on your path to health:

Healthy Eating:

FoodRoutes
Promotes buying fresh local produce.
www.foodroutes.org

Harvest Eating
You'll find wonderful healthy and fresh recipes from Chef Keith Snow.
www.harvesteating.com

Local Harvest
Connecting you to your local sustainable farms, farmer's markets, and organic restaurants though their on-line search.
www.localharvest.org

Produce for Better Health Foundation
You'll find excellent information and simple ways to add more fruits and vegetables to every eating occasion.
www.fruitsandveggiesmorematters.org

Sustainable Table
Celebrates the sustainable food movement, educates consumers on food-related issues and works to build community through food.
www.sustainabletable.org

The Worlds Healthiest Foods
Contains excellent information about healthy eating and cooking.
www.whfoods.org

Vital Choice
High quality wild harvest seafood.
www.vitalchoice.com

Wholesome Harvest
A coalition of over 40 small family farms offering premium organic certified poultry and meats to grocers, chefs and households.
www.wholesomeharvest.com

General Health:

National Women's Health Information Center (NWHIC)
www.womenshealth.gov

National Osteoporosis Foundation
www.nof.org

Mayo Clinic
A not-for-profit medical practice dedicated to the diagnosis and treatment of virtually every type of complex illness.
www.mayoclinic.com

The American Dietetic Association
www.eatright.org

American Institute for Cancer Research
An excellent resource to learn about cancer preventing foods.
www.aicr.org

Fitness:

America On the Move
A national program dedicated to helping individuals and communities improve their lives through healthy eating and active living.
www.americaonthemove.org

Shape Up America!
A national foundation with information on healthy weight management.
www.shapeup.org

Small Step
Straight forward information on improving health, nutrition, and physical activity.
www.smallstep.gov

Yoga Journal
Learn about the benefits of yoga and how to integrate yoga into your life.
www.yogajournal.com

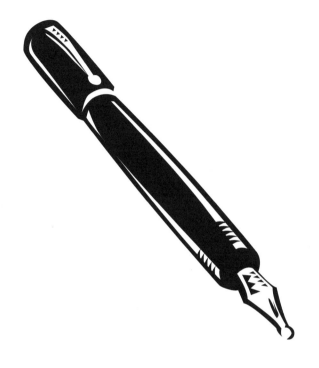

Forms

Food Journal - 1

	Foods Eaten	Record Degree of Hunger 1-10 And Mood	Nutritional Value
Breakfast		Hunger_____ Angry Content Depressed Frustrated Happy Sad Stressed Tired	Low Medium High
Lunch		Hunger_____ Angry Content Depressed Frustrated Happy Sad Stressed Tired	Low Medium High
Dinner		Hunger_____ Angry Content Depressed Frustrated Happy Sad Stressed Tired	Low Medium High
Snacks		Angry Anxious Depressed Feeling Empty Habit Just Because Lonely Other Stimulus Reward Being Sociable Stressed TV Ad	Low Medium High

Food Journal - 2

Foods Eaten	Record Degree of Hunger 1-10 And Mood	Nutritional Value
Breakfast	Hunger_____ Angry Content Depressed Frustrated Happy Sad Stressed Tired	Low Medium High
Lunch	Hunger_____ Angry Content Depressed Frustrated Happy Sad Stressed Tired	Low Medium High
Dinner	Hunger_____ Angry Content Depressed Frustrated Happy Sad Stressed Tired	Low Medium High
Snacks	Angry Anxious Depressed Feeling Empty Habit Just Because Lonely Other Stimulus Reward Being Sociable Stressed TV Ad	Low Medium High

Food Journal - 3

	Foods Eaten	Record Degree of Hunger 1-10 And Mood	Nutritional Value
Breakfast		Hunger_____ Angry Content Depressed Frustrated Happy Sad Stressed Tired	Low Medium High
Lunch		Hunger_____ Angry Content Depressed Frustrated Happy Sad Stressed Tired	Low Medium High
Dinner		Hunger_____ Angry Content Depressed Frustrated Happy Sad Stressed Tired	Low Medium High
Snacks		Angry Anxious Depressed Feeling Empty Habit Just Because Lonely Other Stimulus Reward Being Sociable Stressed TV Ad	Low Medium High

Food Journal - 4

	Foods Eaten	Record Degree of Hunger 1-10 And Mood	Nutritional Value
Breakfast		Hunger_____ Angry Content Depressed Frustrated Happy Sad Stressed Tired	Low Medium High
Lunch		Hunger_____ Angry Content Depressed Frustrated Happy Sad Stressed Tired	Low Medium High
Dinner		Hunger_____ Angry Content Depressed Frustrated Happy Sad Stressed Tired	Low Medium High
Snacks		Angry Anxious Depressed Feeling Empty Habit Just Because Lonely Other Stimulus Reward Being Sociable Stressed TV Ad	Low Medium High

Food Journal - 5

	Foods Eaten	Record Degree of Hunger 1-10 And Mood	Nutritional Value
Breakfast		Hunger_____ Angry Content Depressed Frustrated Happy Sad Stressed Tired	Low Medium High
Lunch		Hunger_____ Angry Content Depressed Frustrated Happy Sad Stressed Tired	Low Medium High
Dinner		Hunger_____ Angry Content Depressed Frustrated Happy Sad Stressed Tired	Low Medium High
Snacks		Angry Anxious Depressed Feeling Empty Habit Just Because Lonely Other Stimulus Reward Being Sociable Stressed TV Ad	Low Medium High

Food Journal - 6

	Foods Eaten	Record Degree of Hunger 1-10 And Mood	Nutritional Value
Breakfast		Hunger_____ Angry Content Depressed Frustrated Happy Sad Stressed Tired	Low Medium High
Lunch		Hunger_____ Angry Content Depressed Frustrated Happy Sad Stressed Tired	Low Medium High
Dinner		Hunger_____ Angry Content Depressed Frustrated Happy Sad Stressed Tired	Low Medium High
Snacks		Angry Anxious Depressed Feeling Empty Habit Just Because Lonely Other Stimulus Reward Being Sociable Stressed TV Ad	Low Medium High

Food Journal - 7

	Foods Eaten	Record Degree of Hunger 1-10 And Mood	Nutritional Value
Breakfast		Hunger_____ Angry Content Depressed Frustrated Happy Sad Stressed Tired	Low Medium High
Lunch		Hunger_____ Angry Content Depressed Frustrated Happy Sad Stressed Tired	Low Medium High
Dinner		Hunger_____ Angry Content Depressed Frustrated Happy Sad Stressed Tired	Low Medium High
Snacks		Angry Anxious Depressed Feeling Empty Habit Just Because Lonely Other Stimulus Reward Being Sociable Stressed TV Ad	Low Medium High

Emotional Eating Diary

Day of Week _____ Time _____ **Food Wanted** _____

Is this food really necessary? YES ___ NO ___

How long has it been since you last ate? _____

Why do you want this particular food?

Look ___ Smell ___ Taste ___ Feel ___ Other ___

What emotional need or feeling are you trying to satisfy? _____

What are your thoughts at this time? _____

What triggered this need for food? Could you satisfy your need in another way? YES ___ NO ___
How? _____

Did you eat to satisfy an emotional rather than a physical need? YES ___ NO ___
If yes, why did you eat? _____

How could you change that response in the future? _____
_____

Did food satisfy your need? YES ___ NO ___
If no, why not? _____

Emotional Eating Diary

Day of Week _____ Time _____ **Food Wanted** _____

Is this food really necessary? YES ___ NO ___

How long has it been since you last ate? _____

Why do you want this particular food?
Look ___ Smell ___ Taste ___ Feel ___ Other ___

What emotional need or feeling are you trying to satisfy? _____

What are your thoughts at this time? _____

What triggered this need for food? Could you satisfy your need in another way? YES ___ NO ___
How? _____

Did you eat to satisfy an emotional rather than a physical need? YES ___ NO ___
If yes, why did you eat? _____

How could you change that response in the future? _____
_____

Did food satisfy your need? YES ___ NO ___
If no, why not? _____

RESPONSE

AFFIRMATION

Affirmation Response Exercise

RESPONSE

AFFIRMATION

*Be proud of yourself for finally making this journey and
continue to practice what you have learned.*

*Be secure in the knowledge that the insights and changes you
are making will resonate through the rest of your life.*

*True freedom is yours, dance through life and share your personal discoveries
with friends, family, and the people who need your encouragement.*

And always remember to share your joy with the world!

*Check our web site at **www.bodyesteem.com** for useful tools, helpful hints, and the
latest healthy weight loss discoveries. You'll also find a community of woman who are
always there to reach out to for help, encouragement, and sharing.*

Additional Instructions Regarding the Recordings

I am acutely aware that you are probably overwhelmed with just your daily activities and trying to fit time for this program into your daily schedule may seem like the "straw that could break the camel's back".

If you are unable to do the reading and/or written exercises on a daily basis, listening to one of the recordings is an alternative you will find very beneficial on a number of levels. I'm not saying that you should not do the reading and the written exercises - they are an integral part of your being successful in reaching your weight goal. What I am saying is . . . just do what you comfortably can each day . . . and if you can only do one thing . . . listen to one of the recorded programs. If you don't have the time during the day, then listen at night as you go to sleep. Listening to them repeatedly will reinforce the suggestions and create positive changes at your subconscious level of awareness.

The following schedule will allow you to receive the maximum results:

CD #1

Track 1 - *Let's Make An Agreement* – Listen to this recording for 14 to 21 days.
You should feel your motivation and commitment to reaching your goal increasing.

Track 2 - *Imaging Positive Results* – Listen to this recording for 14 to 21 days.
You should begin to feel a desire to exercise on a daily basis. You will also begin to look at food in a different way. You will find yourself choosing foods for their nutritional value as you eat less and enjoy it more.

Track 3 - *Set Yourself Free* – This recording will help you release negative emotions you may be suppressing. The recording is initially to be used after completing "Mental Exercise 4" and the "Suppressed Anger" exercise in the Taking Action section. After you have completed those exercises you may continue to listen to it periodically until you feel you have released all of your suppressed emotions.

Continue to listen to the *Let's Make an Agreement* and *Imaging Positive Results* recordings, for another 7 – 10 days, alternating them on a daily basis.

Track 4 - *Adventure in Self-Love* – This recording is introduced in the Self Reflections – Self-Love section of this book. Listen to this recording for 4 days then alternate with Recordings 1 thru 3 for another 10 days.

CD #2

Track 1 - *The New You* - As you listen to this recording you will create your future reality. You will create a mental picture of the physical image that is perfect for you. Listen to this recording for 14 to 21 days, periodically alternating with any of the programs on CD #1.

Track 2 - *Eliminating Stress* - This recording will help you release stress and also deal with stress in a more positive way in your daily life. You may listen to this recording if you have had a particularly stressful day or when you go to sleep at night.

Track 3 - *Mental Exercises* - This recording is designed to only be used with the Mental Exercises in each section. It is designed to help you uncover the deeper issues that may be contributing to your overweight. Uncovering and resolving these issues will insure that your weight loss efforts will be successful and permanent.